Making Safe Food

Making safe food:
A management guide for
microbiological quality

W. F. Harrigan & R. W. A. Park

University of Reading, UK

ACADEMIC PRESS
Harcourt Brace Jovanovich, Publishers
London   San Diego   New York   Boston
Sydney   Tokyo   Toronto

ACADEMIC PRESS LIMITED
24–28 Oval Road
London NW1 7DX

United States Edition published by
ACADEMIC PRESS INC.
San Diego, CA 92101

This book is printed on acid-free paper
A catalogue record for this book is available from the British Library
ISBN 0-12-326045-0

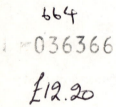
Typeset in Imprint by Photo·graphics, Honiton, Devon
Printed and bound in Great Britain by Mackays of Chatham PLC
Chatham, Kent

Contents

To those who care

Preface

Yoghurt is a safe food – or so we thought until the summer of 1989, when 27 people throughout northern England and Wales suffered from botulism after consuming hazelnut yoghurt that had been manufactured using a canned hazelnut purée which had received an insufficient heat-treatment. Eight of the 27 required life-support, and one died. In 1985 within a 2-week period, approximately 18 000 people in northern Illinois contracted salmonella enteritis from milk that had been pasteurized and subsequently contaminated by raw milk through a faulty valve. During November and early December 1985, 26 babies in England and Wales caught salmonella enteritis, apparently from being fed milk prepared from dried-milk powder from one particular factory. One of the babies died. All remaining products were recalled by the factory, which eventually closed with a financial loss of several million pounds. In 1978, a man and wife invited a brother and sister-in-law for a meal which included salmon from a can. All four were taken severely ill with botulism and were put on life-support machines, but two died of the illness.

All this suffering was caused because of some shortcoming at some stage during the preparation of the food that these people ate. Unfortunately food-related diseases are extremely common throughout the world, even though knowledge exists to prevent them.

This book has been written to assist those concerned with the production, distribution and sale of food, in whose hands lies responsibility for making and selling safe food. There are already published detailed manuals that provide descriptions of laboratory methodology, acceptance sampling plans and the like (e.g. ICMSF, 1978, 1980, 1986, 1988; Harrigan & McCance, 1976). However, there is a large gulf between the quality management books, read and understood by people with a management and business-studies orientation on the one hand, and the food microbiology and food hygiene books, read and understood by food scientists, food technologists and microbiologists, on the other. This book is an attempt to bridge that gulf, so that the management-oriented can understand some of the strengths and weaknesses of the current practices in food microbiology, and food microbiologists can apply their science more realistically and effectively in the production and distribution system.

We present various principles of food microbiology and processing, and include: legislation; design and management of microbiological laboratories; and the interpretation of results. Legislation must be considered by anyone offering food for sale; a badly designed and run microbiology laboratory can be a serious hazard; and results are only as good as the level of informed consideration they receive. Ever conscious of the vast amount of work undertaken by the more enlightened companies in the food industry, by workers in research institutes, government establishments, universities and other institutes of higher education, and the wealth of literature available, we have aimed at being concise. Few references have been given in the text; the worker seriously concerned to follow up the points made will want to get involved in detailed study, using specialist books, reviews and original scientific papers, including those we list in the bibliography.

We wish to thank our fellow microbiologists and food scientists who have contributed knowledge of these subjects, which we have gained over 35 years, either through lectures and discussions, or through their contributions to the world's literature, on which we have drawn. We also thank Ms Gina Fullerlove of Academic Press, and our wives, Rita and Angela, for their encouragement to us in producing this book.

W.F. Harrigan
Department of Food Science
and Technology
University of Reading
Whiteknights
P O Box 226
Reading RG6 2AP
_UK_

R.W.A. Park
Department of Microbiology
University of Reading
Whiteknights
P O Box 228
Reading
_RG6 2AJ_
_UK_

1
Microorganisms and food

1.1 The nature of microorganisms

The term 'microorganism' is generally applied to any single-celled organism, or organism consisting of cells that show little or no differentiation. In practice this means that the groups of microorganisms are: the prokaryotes – bacteria and cyanobacteria; the protists – fungi, protozoa and algae; viruses and prions. Parasitic animals are not included within the microorganisms and will be considered only occasionally in this book, but they are very important in human disease and must not be overlooked in the context of food quality. Though all microbes are small, the range of sizes is enormous. The largest protozoon is more than 10 000 times the length of the smallest virus – a size ratio similar to that of a 10-storey building to an ant.

1.2 Some characteristics of bacteria

Bacterial cells are usually less than 1 μm wide and 5 μm long. A solid mass of bacteria 1 cm^3 comprises about 10^{12} cells. An apparently clear liquid may contain 10^5 bacteria per cubic centimetre, the surface of spoilt red meat 10^9 per square centimetre, and a dense liquid culture a similar number per cubic centimetre. Bacteria are prokaryotes and so they have a much simpler internal structure than fungi and other eukaryotes; nonetheless they have several interesting structural features (Fig. 1.1). They reproduce asexually by binary fission, sometimes as quickly as every 15 minutes. There are many kinds of bacteria, which can be distinguished from one another by using one or more of a

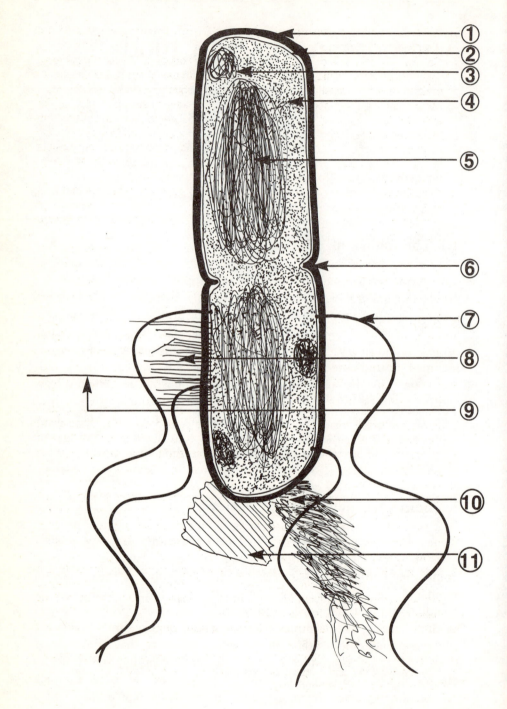

Figure 1.1 A typical bacterium (0.7 μm × 2.5 μm). (Structures marked* are not possessed by all bacteria.)

1. *Cell wall.* A structure of which 'murein', a framework of polysaccharides cross-linked by peptides, is the substance giving strength and shape to the bacterium. In Gram-positive bacteria the cell wall appears uniform, with murein the main component. In Gram-negative bacteria, murein constitutes about 10% of the wall. Outside the murein is a lipoprotein and lipopolysaccharide layer called the 'outer membrane'. The region between the outer membrane and the cyloplasmic membrane contains the murein and is called the 'periplasm' or 'periplasmic space'. The cell wall antigens are important for identifying some bacteria (e.g. the 'O' antigens of *Salmonella* spp.) and in interactions with hosts.

2. *Cytoplasmic membrane.* The lipoprotein structure bounding the cytoplasm. It is the site of attachment of flagella and fimbriae; it regulates passage of substances into and out of the cell, and it is crucially involved in the energy state of the cell.

3. *Plasmid*.* A usually inessential piece of double helical DNA, much smaller than the chromosome. It replicates independently of the chromosome (autonomous state) or may become integrated into it (integrated state).

4. *Cytoplasm.* Contains ribosomes (involved in protein synthesis) and the many other components involved in the metabolism of the cell.

5. *Bacterial chromosome.* A piece of double helical DNA about 1 mm long, in the form of a closed circle folded on itself many times. It is much simpler in structure than are the chromosomes of eukaryote cells (protozoa, fungi, algae, plants and animals).

6. *Developing cross wall.* To separate from each other the two new cells being formed by the previously single cell.

7. *Flagellum** (plural: flagella). A rigid helical structure of globular protein molecules which rotates from the base that is embedded in the cytoplasmic membrane. It is responsible for motility of the bacterium and for the flagellar antigens (e.g. the 'H' antigens of *Salmonella* spp.), that can be used in identification. Flagella can occur only at one or both ends of the bacterium ('polar flagellation') or all round the bacterium ('peritrichous flagellation').

8. *Common fimbria** (plural: fimbriae, also called common pilus – plural: pili). A straight rigid structure of globular protein molecules, originating from the cytoplasmic membrane, responsible for attaching the bacterium to surfaces (e.g. of the gut wall or pipes circulating water in industrial plant). The cell may have hundreds of common fimbriae.

9. *Sex fimbria** (plural: fimbriae, also called sex pilus – plural: pili). Similar to, but longer than, common fimbriae and responsible for conjugation in some bacteria, resulting in transfer of DNA from a donor to a recipient organism. The cell will have not more than a few sex fimbriae.

10. *Slime layer*.* Material, usually polysaccharide, produced by the cell and remaining only loosely associated with it.

11. *Capsule*.* A distinct structure, unlike a slime layer, usually of polysaccharide, surrounding the cell. It may confer resistance to host defence mechanisms and so be important in pathogenicity.

variety of features (including morphology, reaction in Gram's staining method, behaviour in physiological and biochemical tests, chemical composition of walls and membranes, base sequence of the RNA in ribosomes, G+C ratio of the DNA, serological reactions, and sensitivity to different bacteriophages). There are important differences between bacteria with regard to nutritional requirements and response to various environmental factors.

1.2.1 Nutrition

Some bacteria require no organic compounds and may even be inhibited by them, but such bacteria are not of importance in connection with food. Most bacteria are heterotrophs – they need organic material for growth. Some need only one organic compound and mineral salts, some need a fermentable carbohydrate, some need one or more specific organic compounds such as particular amino acids and/or vitamins as well as an organic energy source, and some require a wide range of compounds, a few even being unable to reproduce outside a living host cell. The minimum nutritional requirements of bacteria are not necessarily closely linked to their normal habitat. For example many salmonellae, which cause enteritis, can grow in a simple mineral-salts medium that contains glucose as carbon and energy source and ammonium ion as nitrogen source.

1.2.2 Gaseous requirements

Some bacteria, the obligate aerobes, must have oxygen and can grow only in the presence of air. Some, the microaerophiles, require oxygen, but die, or at least will not grow, unless the concentration is much lower than in air. Two categories can grow in both the presence and absence of oxygen. One of these (the facultative anaerobes) grows better in the presence of oxygen than in its absence. The other (the aerotolerant anaerobes) does not benefit from oxygen. Often the term facultative anaerobe is used for both of these groups. The obligate anaerobes are sensitive to oxygen. Some obligate anaerobes are extremely intolerant of oxygen, and will die if exposed to it for even a short time; others show some tolerance and are able to grow as long as the concentration is low. The oxidation–reduction potential (E_h value) of the environment is often crucial to survival and growth. It is affected by the availability of oxygen and the number and nature of the oxidation–reduction systems present.

Carbon dioxide at a concentration above that normally present in air is required by some bacteria, called capnophiles. However, all bacteria require some CO_2; growth can be suspended indefinitely by removing and excluding the gas from the environment. Many obligate aerobes are inhibited by high concentrations of CO_2.

1.2.3 Temperature

Microbial growth can occur from less than $-20°C$ to over $90°C$, but no one organism can grow over this whole range. Two types of organisms with respect to growth at low temperature are recognized: psychrophiles, which have an optimum growth temperature below $20°C$; and psychrotrophs, which can grow at low temperatures but have an optimum growth temperature above $20°C$. Psychrotrophs are more important than psychrophiles in the food industry, because of their flexibility with respect to temperature. Psychrophiles are readily killed by temperatures only slightly in excess of $20°C$. Mesophiles, some of which are also psychrotrophs, grow best in the region $20–45°C$, and include the human pathogens. Thermophiles cannot grow below about $45°C$. All these categories relate to the ability of the organism to *grow* at the temperature indicated; they do not relate directly to heat resistance. The term 'thermoduric' means that an organism can *survive* at high temperature; it says nothing about the temperature required for growth. Endospores, produced by *Bacillus* and *Clostridium*, are resting stages that are particularly resistant to heat and they are therefore of crucial importance in the canning industry. (Some species of *Bacillus* are thermoduric, psychrotrophic mesophiles!)

1.2.4 Water

Water is the largest component of bacterial cells, as it is of all other life. For bacteria to be able to grow there must be a plentiful supply of water, both to serve as a component and for the transport of metabolites. For most bacteria, the concentration of solutes (e.g. sodium chloride, sucrose) in the external environment must be low, otherwise the attraction of the solute for the water molecules restricts the ability of the organisms to take up water for growth.

1.2.5 pH value and buffering capacity

The pH value of the bacterial environment profoundly affects many aspects of growth and survival. Most bacteria are considered to prefer a slightly alkaline pH value, but some important food bacteria, for example *Lactobacillus* and *Acetobacter*, thrive under acidic conditions. It is important to remember, particularly in understanding the inhibitory nature of weak acids (e.g. nitrous acid, sulphurous acid, benzoic acid) at different pH values, that a change of one unit of pH value represents a 10-fold change in hydrogen ion concentration. The ability of particular bacteria to change the pH value of a food will depend on the buffering capacity of the food (usually greatest in high-protein foods), the availability of a substrate that can be metabolized to products which will change the pH value, and the pK values of the products. These factors can play an important part in food safety and the detection of pathogens. For example, it is possible for *Staphylococcus aureus* to grow and produce toxin in milk to be used for cheese before a weak starter culture has fermented the lactose sufficiently to lower the pH value. When the pH value is eventually lowered the *S. aureus* will be killed but the toxin will remain in the cheese and give rise to intoxications, even though, of course, the causative organism cannot be detected on cultivation of the cheese. Thoughtless suspension of samples of dried products in unbuffered diluent during laboratory investigations can kill organisms if acid results.

1.2.6 Inhibitory substances

Many substances are inhibitory to bacteria. Some of these are used as disinfectants for industrial plant, work surfaces, etc. A few are used as preservatives in food and in other products. Bacteria often differ from one another in their resistance to a particular agent and use is made of this in the devising of selective and enrichment media for the isolation of certain types of bacteria in the presence of other types. Differences can be phenotypic as well as genetic. Thus one may add a selective inhibitor to a medium for the selective isolation of *Salmonella* bacteria, because it has been found in laboratory tests using healthy salmonellae that the organisms are not affected by the concentration used, whereas bacteria of other genera are. However, salmonellae from dried or frozen products may be in such a damaged state that they will themselves be unable to resist the inhibitor, and so give a false negative result.

1.2.7 *The phases of growth in a batch culture*

When a bacterium is inoculated into a fresh liquid medium some time elapses before it multiplies. This period, called the lag phase, is when spores germinate, nutrients are taken up, new enzymes are formed to metabolize the fresh medium, and so on. Then multiplication occurs and the culture is said to be in the logarithmic (log) phase or exponential phase. The number of bacteria being produced is proportional to the number present, each bacterium reproducing itself. Note that the *proportional* increase with time is the same throughout the log phase – the doubling time is constant, but the *number* produced in a given time depends on the number present. Consequently a clean food takes much longer to spoil than one which has been heavily contaminated. After a while growth ceases, either because one crucial nutrient has been depleted or because toxic metabolites have accumulated, and the culture is said to be in the stationary phase – the numbers neither increasing nor decreasing. Eventually the population dies, the number dying being proportional to the number alive at the time, this stage being called the death phase or decline phase. It is possible to keep organisms growing continually by using chemostat or turbidostat continuous-culture apparatus and such procedures resemble certain natural situations (but not growth on, or in, food) more closely than do batch cultures. The simple batch-culture situation is not seen when bacteria are on solid media because diffusion gradients of nutrients and of waste products cause heterogeneity in the population.

1.3 The fungi

The moulds and yeasts, which are the most important fungi in the context of food hygiene, are larger than bacteria and structurally more complex, being typical eukaryotes in having mitochondria, Golgi apparatus, distinct nuclei with true chromosomes, and so on. Yeasts exist as single cells or short chains and reproduce by budding or fission. They have a diameter of 4 μm or more. Thus one yeast cell has the same volume and hence biomass as 60 or more typical bacteria. Moulds grow as a mycelium consisting of a complex array of tubes called hyphae, of indefinite length and from about 4 to 20 μm in diameter. Their spread throughout the environment is achieved principally by the production of large numbers of spores or conidia. Thus, whereas for bacteria and yeasts, number gives a reasonable indication of the amount of contamination of a food, the number of mould colony-forming units has very little relationship to the amount of contamination by moulds.

Environmental factors have similar effects on moulds and yeasts as on bacteria but there are important differences. Thus, moulds and yeasts tend to prefer acid pH values and to be capable of growth at lower water activity values than bacteria. The resting stages produced by fungi tend not to be resistant to heat but in very acid foods, such as canned fruit, the most resistant life form of consequence can often be the spores of the mould *Byssochlamys fulva*, which can survive processing and subsequently spoil the product.

1.4 Protozoa, algae, viruses and prions

These microorganisms do not grow on food and so the only aspects of importance are their pathogenicity or toxigenicity and their resistance to various processing procedures. Many are more sensitive than the average vegetative bacterium but there are some important exceptions. Protozoa have a similar structure to animal cells although they sometimes form resting stages which may cause trouble by being resistant to disinfectants, particularly chlorine as used in the water industry. Algae can be thought of as simple plants in that they carry out photosynthesis, evolving oxgyen, and they have the green pigment, chlorophyll, for capturing the light energy they use. However, not all algae are green, because they have other pigments which may mask the green colour.

Viruses consist of only one type of nucleic acid in a more or less complex enclosure. Some can be cultivated in hen eggs or tissue culture, but detection and study is much more complex and expensive than is the case with bacteria. They have a life cycle which consists of the particulate, non-replicative phase, by which they pass from one cell or organism to another as structures of 20–300 nm; and the replicative phase, when they are in the host cell in the form of nucleic acid and not recognizable as a distinct entity. Many viruses are important in the food industry because of their pathogenicity for human beings via the faecal–oral route (Section 2.2). Viruses that attack bacteria (i.e. 'bacteriophages' or 'phages') are important in at least three ways. Some cause great damage by attacking bacteria used as starter cultures in the manufacture of cheese, etc. Secondly, some bacteriophages are used in genetic engineering to transfer genes from one strain of bacterium to another by the process of transduction. Thirdly, bacteriophages are used in 'phage typing', which is a simple means of making fine distinctions between strains of bacteria that appear identical by other tests. A collection of reference phages which each attack a different range of strains of the species of interest is made. Any new strain is then tested for its pattern of sensitivity against the collection to give its 'phage type' (PT). Phage typing is especially useful in tracing the source of a particular strain of *Staphylococcus aureus* or of certain *Salmonella* species involved in outbreaks of food-related diseases.

The structure of prions, the agents of the sheep disease scrapie and the cattle disease bovine spongiform encephalopathy, is something of a mystery but we know that the agents are at least predominantly protein. They are extremely resistant to heat.

1.5 The relevance of microorganisms to the food industry

Microorganisms are involved in several processes which enhance the quality of our food (e.g. in manufacture of foods – cheese, yoghurt, fermented fish and meat products, soy sauce, bread, wine, tempeh; in production of food additives – vinegar, citric acid, sodium glutamate, pigments; as sources of enzymes for processing – rennin substitutes, pectinase) and as foods in their own right – for example, mushrooms, yeast extract and mycoprotein. Their positive contributions should not be overlooked. However, this book is concerned chiefly with the problems that microorganisms can cause in the food industry by reducing the quality of foods, and with ways to solve these problems.

1.6 Deleterious effects of microorganisms on food

Microorganisms can reduce the quality of foods in various ways, which will be examined in detail in the next four chapters. They can change the food organoleptically so as to deter the potential consumer, or they can make it capable of causing disease. There is no doubt that food-related disease is extremely important throughout the world. In England

and Wales over 60 000 cases are recorded annually, a number which is thought to be only one-tenth or one-hundredth of the actual number of people in these countries who suffer from disease contracted from food. The vast majority of cases are thought to go unrecorded for various reasons – because sufferers do not report their illness to their doctor, or their doctor does not send a sample for analysis, or analysis fails to reveal the causative organism. Thus, one should recognize that in a developed country such as the UK in any one year as much as 10 % of the population will suffer from a food-related disease, and some deaths will result, usually amongst the most vulnerable – the young and the infirm. In developing countries the situation is less clear because of less well-developed diagnostic and reporting facilities, and because of the demand on limited medical facilities by sufferers of a variety of life-threatening diseases. However, it is known that throughout the world in any one year millions of young children die as a result of diarrhoea, much of which has been caused by organisms contracted from water or food.

Unfortunately, various authorities differ over the definitions they give for some of the terms commonly used for microbial diseases associated with foods. In this book we use the term *food-related disease* for any disease that arises because consumed food was contaminated by microorganisms or their metabolites, and we recognize three classes of such diseases. The term *foodborne disease* is used for any disease that arises from the contamination of food by disease-producing agents that cannot multiply, or at any rate have not multiplied, on or in the incriminated food. Such diseases are distinct from *food poisoning*, which we define as any disease that results because microorganisms have *grown* on the food to produce either a sufficiently large population to constitute an infective dose (*infection-type food poisoning*) or the production of a toxin in the food (*intoxication-type food poisoning*). The main discrepancy in nomenclature of these various classes of food-related diseases arises because some authorities use the term 'foodborne disease' to cover both what we have defined as 'foodborne disease' and 'infection-type food poisoning'. They use this broad definition because they recognize that some food-related diseases that usually arise because the causative microorganism has grown on the food, of which salmonella enteritis is perhaps the best example, may arise without the agent having grown on the food. This may happen because the particular food carrying the organism offers protection from the stomach acid, because contamination is very great, or because the consumer is particularly vulnerable. However, such authorities fail to make sufficiently clear what we regard as a crucially important feature, namely that diseases which arise because organisms have grown on the food are at least partly due to improper storage of the food at some stage, whereas those that arise without growth are not.

2
Some foodborne diseases

2.1 The range of foodborne diseases

Potentially, many diseases can be transferred via food from one human being or animal to another human being without the organism having grown on the food to increase its number. It is not possible to draw a clear distinction between this means of spread (to give rise to a 'foodborne disease') and means of spread which require growth on the food to occur (to give rise to an 'infection-type food poisoning'), because the nature of the food, the amount of initial contamination of the food and the sensitivity of the individual eating the food may all affect the outcome. However, some disease-causing organisms are thought never, or only rarely, to be capable of growth on foods. It is these types that will concern us in this chapter and we will consider some of the potentially more common ones. Refrigeration of food infected with such organisms will not necessarily reduce the risk of infection – the organisms may not be adversely affected by such treatment and so the food will remain infective, in some cases more so than if storage had been at room temperature because competing microbes will not grow so fast, and degenerative processes will not be so rapid, at the lower temperature. In fact, the spread of such infections via food can be stopped only by ensuring that the causative organisms do not gain access to the food or that they are killed in, or removed from, the food.

2.2 Viruses

Every virus is essentially a message in a packet and is reproduced only if the message can be inserted into an appropriate living cell. Viruses are moderately to extremely specific about the species of organism and the types of cells they invade. It follows that viruses pathogenic for human beings do not increase in numbers on food nor can they be detected by using artificial media of the types used for bacteria. Some can be detected by cultivation in fertilized hen eggs or in tissue culture of animal cells of particular types, but for several viruses involved in gastroenteritis the only methods of detection at present available involve serology and/or electron microscopy. In some cases the presence of viruses on foods is revealed by epidemiological studies of the people who become ill after eating the food. Some viral diseases are known to be spread by the faecal–oral route, but the extent to which food may be an intermediary in this means of spread is not known. Viruses that are spread by the faecal–oral route usually infect their victims via cells lining the digestive tract (the primary tropism). Some cause gastroenteritis which may be confused with gastroenteritis caused by bacteria, but others may cause no symptoms at this point but be transferred via the lymph or the blood to other tissues (such as nervous tissue) where they may give rise to the symptoms of the disease (the secondary tropism).

Transmission of viruses that cause gastrointestinal diseases may occur by an aerosol from, or direct contact with, an infected human being, or by such a person handling foods or polluting water used for drinking or for preparing foods. Filter-feeding shellfish (molluscs) harvested from sewage-polluted water can be particularly important, as in the case of some bacterial infections, because they concentrate the viruses, probably taken in from sewage-polluted water, and are often eaten without being heated.

Members of the genus *Enterovirus* include some of the best known viruses that are spread by the faecal–oral route. Poliovirus (which causes gastrointestinal symptoms, fever, and, in a few cases, paralysis) can be spread by milk and water; effective vaccination is available and widely used. Coxsackieviruses, echoviruses, and enteroviruses cause a variety of diseases, some severe. However they are responsible for relatively few of the cases of viral gastroenteritis; infection by some of the viruses is not known to give rise to *any* clinical symptoms. Hepatitis A virus, which causes so-called infectious hepatitis, is classified as *Enterovirus* 72. It is spread via the faecal–oral route and has been associated with several well-documented outbreaks involving food, particularly shellfish, or water. It is resistant to chlorine and is a very stable virus. Incubation times can be longer than a month, making epidemiological studies particularly difficult. Some viruses besides Hepatitis virus type A cause hepatitis, but, with the exception of Hepatitis virus type B (which is spread by intimate contact or blood transfusions, etc.), little is known of their relevance.

The genus *Rotavirus* is of considerable importance because members cause many sporadic cases of severe acute diarrhoea and fever, often accompanied by vomiting. The disease is seen particularly in babies and young children – in fact rotaviruses are thought to be responsible for 5 million infant deaths per annum world wide. Caliciviruses, astroviruses and coronaviruses are other types of viruses that cause gastrointestinal disease mainly in babies and young children. Symptoms are similar to, and in some cases less severe than, those caused by rotaviruses.

Adenoviruses are usually associated with acute respiratory diseases but some (particularly the ones difficult to cultivate – the 'fastidious adenoviruses', types 40 and 41) can cause acute gastroenteritis, chiefly in babies and young children, and can be spread by the faecal–oral route. They are probably the next most important causes of infantile gastroenteritis after rotaviruses.

Norwalk virus and several other viruses with similar structure and pathogenicity are known as 'small round structured viruses' or SRSVs. They cause predominantly nausea and vomiting (but also with diarrhoea, fever and abdominal pain), lasting for 1–2 days. Unlike rotaviruses and adenoviruses these cause epidemics, rather than sporadic cases, and occur usually in school children and adults, rather than in infants. They have never been cultivated in the laboratory and so knowledge has been derived from analysis of particles harvested from vomit and faeces of patients. They are relatively resistant to acids and to typical pasteurization treatments. They seem to be the major causes of epidemics of viral gastroenteritis, outbreaks having been associated with water supplies, oysters, salads, etc.

Encephalitis can be spread via the milk from animals, particularly goats, infected with tickborne encephalitis viruses.

2.3 The rickettsiae

Rickettsiae are small bacteria that have never been cultivated in artificial media. They differ from viruses in having both DNA and RNA, and in possessing several structural features of bacteria. The agent of Q (for query) fever, *Coxiella burnetii*, is the only one of importance in connection with food. It causes severe headache and fever and can be spread by drinking milk from an infected cow. The agent shows considerable resistance to heat, a property that has been claimed to be associated with the production of heat-resistant endospores, and so it may occur in pasteurized milk.

2.4 Prions

Prions are unusual transmissible pathogens causing degenerative diseases of the central nervous system in animals and human beings. Kuru, a disease seen in some human cannibals that eat the brains of infected relatives, is the only known example, albeit a bizarre one, of a foodborne prion infection of human beings. Until recently, the best known disease caused by these agents in animals was scrapie, which occurs in sheep. However, a similar disease has developed in cattle, bovine spongiform encephalopathy, which is also caused by a prion, and infections in several other species have been reported. The possibility that such agents might spread from food animals to human beings is now being seriously considered and is giving rise to some concern. Prions are very resistant to heat, more so than the most resistant bacterial endospores, and are composed largely, or entirely, of an abnormal form of protein from the host. No prion-specific nucleic acid is known to be required for transmission of the diseases. Control is by ensuring that no infectious material, usually taken to be only nervous tissue from an infected animal, is passed to another animal or to a human being, but the extent of precautions required is the subject of scientific research and vigorous public debate.

2.5 Protozoa and parasites

Giardia, *Cryptosporidium*, *Balantidium*, *Entamoeba*, some other protozoa, and various parasites such as tapeworms, hookworms, roundworms and flukes can be transmitted by infected water and possibly food. Sources may be other infected human beings, who may not themselves show clinical signs of the infection, or, in certain cases, animals. Some species have resistant forms which survive for weeks in the environment and are resistant to normally used concentrations of chlorine in water

supplies. Some infections cause symptoms that can be confused with
bacterial enteritis, and transmission is often by the faecal–oral route,
the use of human sewage to fertilize salad crops facilitating spread.

2.6 Foodborne bacteria that cause diseases that do not involve gastroenteritis

In some cases food produced from diseased animals will be the source
of infection for various bacterial diseases. Examples are tuberculosis
(*Mycobacterium bovis* and *M. tuberculosis*), brucellosis (*Brucella
abortus* – cattle; *Brucella melitensis* – goats); and listeriosis (*Listeria
monocytogenes*, see Section 4.3). In these cases milk, or occasionally
meat, will be the vehicle. Milk can also become contaminated by release
of bacteria from infected but healthy animals (e.g. *Corynebacterium
diphtheriae*, which causes diphtheria, can enter the milk during milking
from small infected lesions on the cow teat). Alternatively, contamination
at or after milking can occur from human carriers or domestic or wild
animals. In all these cases control can be effected by avoiding cross
contamination, by pasteurization of milk, and, in some cases, by
eradication of the disease from the animals.

2.7 Foodborne bacteria that cause gastroenteritis

Many of the bacteria that cause gastroenteritis are capable of growing
on various foods under commonly used holding conditions. Such
bacteria include *Salmonella* spp., *Shigella* spp., *Vibrio cholerae* and
Escherichia coli. Sometimes food will be so heavily contaminated as to
contain a sufficiently large number of these organisms to cause disease
so that further growth is not required, or the food will be of a type
that protects the organisms from the acid barrier of the stomach so
that a smaller dose than usual is infective. Alternatively, the organisms
may require only a small number to initiate infection so that growth
on infected food prior to its ingestion is not necessary (*Shigella* can
infect with as few as 100 organisms). These types of bacteria will be
considered in the context of Chapter 4. However, *Campylobacter*
bacteria cannot grow on food, and deserve special consideration here.

2.8 Campylobacteriosis

In developed countries *Campylobacter* is the most commonly recorded cause of infectious diarrhoea, exceeding even *Salmonella*. In developing countries infection in infancy appears to be much more common and so immunity develops early in life, apparently causing there to be no correlation in such countries between infections and diarrhoea in adults. The disease can take the form of a profuse watery diarrhoea ('enteritis'), or severe abdominal pain and bloody diarrhoea ('colitis'). In fact, the term 'enteritis' is often used to cover all types of enteric disease caused by campylobacters. Although the disease can be very debilitating and in some cases last for several weeks it is almost never fatal in developed countries. In developing countries the situation is less clear but infected infants may die.

Campylobacters are present in the gut of poultry, cattle, pigs, sheep, and a variety of wild animals and birds. There are several species, the ones most commonly incriminated in enteritis being *C. jejuni* and *C. coli*. There are many different serovars, and strains vary with respect to the ability to give positive results in different *in vitro* and *in vivo* tests to detect toxin production. However, there seems little evidence of correlation of the results of these tests with pathogenicity; in fact it is prudent to regard any campylobacter as capable of causing enteritis and to take steps to exclude it from food.

Isolation of the organisms is by use of selective media or the use of filters of pore size 0.45 or 0.65 μm, which pass some of the campylobacters but not most of the other bacteria. Incubation has to be in a microaerobic atmosphere, usually one in which oxygen is at a concentration of 5 % or less, because the organisms need oxygen for growth but are inhibited by the concentration found in air. Identity can be confirmed by microscopy and various biochemical tests or by using the Microscreen ® campylobacter serological latex test. The campylobacters incriminated in enteritis cannot grow below 30°C but can grow up to 43°C. They are referred to as 'thermophilic' campylobacters to distinguish them from those with a slightly lower growth-temperature range, even though the organism cannot grow at the high temperatures characteristic of the truly thermophilic bacteria.

Campylobacters are not particularly resistant bacteria. They are sensitive to dehydration, to acids and to even moderate heating, having a D value at 55°C of about 1 minute and a z value of about 5°C. Thus, acidic foods and pasteurized foods are not infectious. Campylobacters survive well at refrigerator temperatures with a decimal reduction time of several days when inoculated on to cooked meat. In the past they have been reported to be particularly sensitive to freezing, but, though injured, many can be recovered if suitable resuscitation techniques are used. Most infections of human beings in developed countries are thought to arise from meat infected with gut contents of the animals at slaughter. If the meat surface is allowed to dry, as is the case with most red meats immediately after slaughter, the numbers of campylobacters fall markedly. However, in the case of chickens slaughtered in modern automated units and packed moist, and in the case of offal, which remains moist, the campylobacters survive well. Thus, chicken is thought to be a major source of campylobacter infection of foods in the kitchen, where it is presumed to be spread to food that will be eaten without further heating. There have been many outbreaks caused by the consumption of raw milk, but it is not clear whether the milk becomes infected by faecal contamination or as a result of mastitis caused by *Campylobacter* spp. Campylobacter mastitis has been reported, but it is very rare, whereas campylobacters are present in large numbers in the faeces of many milking cows. Some outbreaks have been caused by contaminated drinking water. It is surprising that person-to-person spread is extremely rare, particularly as infected faeces can contain 10^8 or more campylobacters per gram and the infective dose may in some circumstances be less than 10^3.

In light of various studies made in developing countries one can expect that, as improvements in hygiene are made, infections in infants there will become rarer, immunity in older children and adults will fall, and the pattern of cases seen at present only in developed countries, where cases are most common in teenagers and adults, will become more widespread.

2.9 Anthrax

Bacillus anthracis, the causative organism of anthrax, has a wide host range, causing disease in cattle and other domestic and wild animals as well as in human beings. When meats or body fluids infected with *Bacillus anthracis* are exposed to air the organism forms heat-resistant endospores. It is possible for human beings to contract intestinal anthrax through eating infected meat and milk. Either a cholera-like gastroenteritis with watery diarrhoea or acute abdominal pain and bloody diarrhoea results, the mortality rate being very high. The serious and infectious nature of anthrax means that all infected animals should be destroyed without a post-mortem being undertaken. Confirmation of infection can be achieved by examination of a small amount of blood, usually from the ear, which will reveal the organism, with the characteristic capsule that it produces when in a host.

3

Intoxication-type food poisoning

3.1 Definition

Intoxication-type food poisoning is defined as being caused by the growth on or in a food of a microorganism producing a metabolite that is toxic to the consumer of that food. Traditionally, the incubation period and symptoms will be such that the link with the causative food can be established by epidemiological investigation, followed by laboratory confirmation. Thus, intoxications caused by *Staphylococcus aureus*, *Clostridium botulinum* and *Bacillus cereus*, for example, are included in national and international statistics on food poisoning, and most authorities would also include scombrotoxicosis and dinoflagellate poisoning. However, food-associated mycotoxicoses such as ergotism, alimentary toxic aleukia, and 'yellow rice disease' are equally examples of intoxication-type food poisoning, but in some mycotoxicoses the incubation period is so long, or the type of disease so often not discernibly associated with food (e.g. hepatoma), that the syndrome is not included in 'food poisoning' statistics.

3.2 Botulism

Although relatively uncommon in most countries, the intoxication gives rise to a neuroparalytic syndrome which is so serious that much of the focus of food processing for the past 60 years has been on destroying or inhibiting *Clostridium botulinum*. The principal foods of concern

Table 3.1 Outbreaks of botulism (adapted from Hauschild, in Doyle, 1989)

Country	Average no. of cases per year*	Fatalities (%)	Food involved† (% outbreaks)				Source (%)	
			Meat	Fish	Vegetable & fruit	Other	Home	Com-mercial
Poland	478	2	87	11	2	0	68	32
China	168	13	10	0	86	4	–	–
Iran	57	11	3	97	0	0	–	–
Italy	48	?	8	8	77	8	–	–
USSR	47	29	17	67	16	0	97	3
W. Germany	42	7	>75	–	–	–	–	–
USA	32	11	14	17	60	9	90	10
France	31	3	86	5	7	2	88	12
Japan	14	23	0	99	1	0	98	2
Canada	11	14	70	22	8	0	97	3
Argentina	7	37	3	10	73	13	77	23
Spain	6	6	42	0	58	0	92	8

* Over various periods mostly between 1970 and 1985.
† In some outbreaks the food remains unidentified.

vary from country to country (Table 3.1). For example, in the USA, home-canned and home-bottled vegetables are important causes of outbreaks. In Japan, botulism is caused primarily by raw and fermented fish products. In the UK, cases of botulism have been rare for many decades, but those that have occurred have been caused by various canned foods or canned components of foods.

Three serovars of *C. botulinum* predominate in human intoxications: Type A (a proteolytic type) and Type B (contains both proteolytic and non-proteolytic strains) are found in soil and water; Type E (a non-proteolytic form) in most parts of the world is primarily aquatic in sediments.

3.2.1 Response to the food environment, and heat resistance

The non-proteolytic strains (especially Type E, with a minimum growth temperature of *c.* 3°C) can give problems in chilled foods even when the 'cold chain' has been maintained. In such foods control of the hazard depends on other environmental parameters such as sodium chloride concentration, a_w, pH, etc. With the increasing demand in many countries for a reduction in salt content, nitrite or other food preservatives, there is a danger of losing the inhibitory control of this organism. Changes in the marketing and retail sectors may also introduce new hazards: for example, prepacking of fresh vegetables such as mushrooms may provide the opportunity for growth of *C. botulinum*.

Many outbreaks of botulism involving the commercial sector, however, are still caused by inadequate attention to hygiene, quality monitoring, or the processing parameters.

3.3 Staphylococcal food poisoning

Staphylococcal food poisoning carries a very low case fatality rate, deaths occurring only in individuals who have other complicating life-threatening factors. However, because of the very short incubation period (as little as 30 minutes before the symptoms show), spectacular outbreaks involving food catering can make the news.

The principal source of the organism is the food handler who is a carrier of an enterotoxigenic strain of *Staphylococcus aureus*. Thus foods commonly incriminated are those which have been handled or manipulated after cooking and which may then be stored above refrigeration temperatures before consumption. The growth of *S. aureus* in a food does not necessarily render the food unacceptable from the point of view of odour or flavour. Cakes and puddings containing whipped cream, custards, mousses, buffet tables with sliced cold meats, vol-au-vents, galantines, etc. all represent major hazards. The more visually attractive the food, the greater the risk, since considerable handling will have been involved and the chef will have displayed his or her art (at ambient temperature!) before the diner is permitted to consume it. It is rare to see 'cold' buffets being set out on refrigerated tables, or even on beds of ice.

Outbreaks occur from time to time in which canned foods such as canned peas are implicated. In these cases the problem usually derives from factory procedures that require the handling of hot cans from the autoclaves to the labelling machines. A human carrier can thus contaminate the outside of the wet can which, whilst still hot, may draw the contaminated liquid into the can through temporary leaks in the can-sealing mastic. However, it *is* possible for enterotoxin to be produced in the food which is to be canned. For example, in an outbreak caused by canned mushrooms, in which the staphylococci were found to have grown and produced enterotoxin in the supplies of plastic-film-wrapped mushrooms used for canning, the heat resistance of the enterotoxin ensured its persistence in the finished product.

The other main source of *S. aureus* is milk from an animal suffering from staphylococcal mastitis. If the organism is permitted to multiply in the milk and to produce toxin, this will then represent a substantial hazard, even in foods which are subsequently heat-treated. Although the bacterium may be killed (a D_{60} of between 2 and 15 minutes, depending on the food), the enterotoxin is relatively heat-stable. Thus, outbreaks of staphylococcal food poisoning have been caused by spray-dried milk in which the staphylococci have been destroyed to undetectably low concentrations by pasteurization and the heating received during the drying process but the enterotoxin has not. Enterotoxin may be present in cheese, resulting from growth of *S. aureus* in the milk before the lactic acid bacteria have lowered the pH sufficiently to kill the organism. Viable *S. aureus* may not be detected in such cheese.

3.4 Food poisoning caused by *Bacillus* species

The most well-known food poisoning species of *Bacillus* is *B. cereus*, but increasingly during recent years, *B. licheniformis* and *B. subtilis* also have been implicated in outbreaks of food poisoning.

Two forms of *B. cereus* food poisoning occur, due to two different types of toxin. One type of food poisoning is an emetic syndrome, with nausea and vomiting occurring 1–5 hours after consumption of the food. Most recorded outbreaks in the UK have been of this type, involving fried or boiled rice in Chinese restaurants or 'take-away' shops. The second type is a diarrhoeal syndrome with an incubation period of 8–16 hours; this is commonly found in eastern European countries involving reheated meat casserole dishes containing large amounts of spices such as paprika and dried pepper added at a late stage in the cooking. Such spices are often heavily contaminated with *Bacillus* spores, which resist the brief exposure to heat and germinate on cooling.

3.5 Mycotoxicoses

A very large number of microfungi produce secondary metabolites that are toxic to humans, and some species produce more than one toxin. Some of the best known are shown in Table 3.2, but other toxigenic fungi commonly found in foods include *Cladosporium*, *Mucor* and *Stachybotrys*.

Reliable assay procedures are available for some specific mycotoxins; for example, aflatoxins can be detected and quantified by TLC, HPLC or ELISA. However, a consumer demand that foods should be screened for *any* (unspecified) mycotoxins is unrealistic because of the great chemical variety of these toxins and the fact that new toxic metabolites are continually being reported. For example, Wood *et al*. (1990) reported a toxic metabolite, walleminol A, produced by *Wallemia sebi*. (*Wallemia sebi* is a common mould on bread and bakery products, and is frequently overlooked in the early stages of its development, for example, on the crust of wholemeal bread, because it produces small, flat, dull, brown colonies.) A protocol for screening for mycotoxins would include bioassay. Animal feeding trials can be undertaken, or pathological changes in chicken embryos can be sought, or, best of all, cytological examination of the effects of food-sample extracts on relevant tissue cultures including human cells can be carried out.

As some mycotoxins are carcinogenic, it is possible that there is no threshold below which there is no effect. This can lead to considerable problems for the law-makers and for government enforcement agencies as analytical techniques become more and more sensitive, because many foods may contain traces of mycotoxins and thus carry a certain risk.

3.6 Shellfish poisoning

Shellfish poisoning (other than that caused by shellfish which is inherently toxic) can take various clinical forms, but in all cases originates from the ingestion of toxin-containing dinoflagellate algae (such as *Gonyaulax* and *Pyrolidinum*) by filter-feeding molluscan shellfish (such as clams and mussels). The dinoflagellates are widely distributed in marine waters, but under certain climatic or other influences their populations may build up to such large numbers that a major public health hazard results from the accumulation of the toxin by shellfish that enter the human food chain. Such outbreaks occur

Table 3.2 Mycotoxins

Name of mycotoxin	Toxigenic organism	Nature of toxic effect
Various ergotoxins	*Claviceps purpurea*	Ergotism, or St Anthony's Fire: pains, convulsions, hallucinations, gangrene of the limbs
Alkaloids	*Ustilago maydis*	Infantile erythroedema (central Europe)
Aflatoxins	*Aspergillus flavus* *A. parasiticus*	? hepatoma, hepatic fibrosis
Islanditoxin, luteoskyrin	*Penicillium islandicum*	'Yellow rice disease'; acute and chronic liver lesions, hepatoma
Sporofusarin, poaefusarin	*Fusarium tricinctum* ('*F. sporotrichioides*')	Alimentary toxic aleukia: frequently fatal. First stage: burning sensations in mouth, gastroenteritis, diarrhoea, vomiting. Second stage if ingestion continues: leucopoenia – reduction in erythrocytes and leucocytes, and granulation of neutrophils. Third stage: angino-haemorrhagia.
Patulin	*Aspergillus clavatus* *Penicillium expansum* *P. patulum*	None known in man (but toxin may be produced in mouldy apples, and will remain active in the pasteurized apple juice)
Ochratoxins	*Aspergillus ochraceus* *A. sulphureus* *Penicillium viridicatum* *P. verrucosum*	Balkan (endemic) nephropathy
?	*Gloeotinia temulenta*	Food poisoning caused by bread made from contaminated rye: giddiness, vertigo, nausea, vomiting, diarrhoea

quite frequently from shellfish from Pacific coastal waters, but shellfish from Atlantic coastal waters are involved rather less frequently.

The gastrointestinal or allergic types of clinical syndrome may be distressing but are usually of relatively short duration, and rarely fatal. However, the paralytic syndrome caused by *Gonyaulax* gonyautoxin and saxitoxin can carry a case fatality rate as high as 10 %.

Avoidance of outbreaks can be effected to some extent by setting up procedures by which coastguard and similar services notify public health and food agencies when 'red tides' or 'algal blooms' have been detected, so that fishing prohibition orders can be issued.

3.7 Scombrotoxic food poisoning

Scombrotoxic food poisoning is caused by microbial spoilage of certain, usually scombroid, species of fish. The fish particularly associated with the intoxication are the various types of tuna (*Thunnus thynnus*, *T. alalunga*, *Euthynnus pelamis*, *Sarda sarda*), mackerel (*Scomber* spp.) and also sardine (*Sardinops sagax*). Spoilage organisms (especially various *Enterobacteriaceae* species) decarboxylate free histidine to produce histamine. Consumption of the histamine gives rise, within a few minutes to a few hours, to symptoms that are analogous to an allergic response – 'flushing' of the face and neck, urticaria, dizziness, and so on. Complete recovery follows in about 12 hours.

4

Infection-type food poisoning

4.1 Definition

An 'infection-type food poisoning' is a disease caused because organisms have multiplied in the food sufficiently to give an infective dose. However, there have been several outbreaks of disease caused by organisms usually associated with infection-type food poisoning (e.g. *Salmonella*) in which multiplication did not appear to have taken place in the food. In such outbreaks the disease is better considered as a foodborne infection (Chapter 2).

4.2 *Salmonella*

There are well over 2000 serovars of *Salmonella*, the majority of which infect a wide range of animals including human beings. A few are more species- or genus-specific; for example *S. typhi* and *S. paratyphi* type A naturally infect only human beings. In any given country, only a small proportion of these 2000 serovars will predominate in the natural environment and in human disease. For example, in the UK in any one year, there are only about 200 that will be environmentally or clinically detected, and only about 10 will feature significantly in human disease.

Two principal types of disease can be caused in human beings – (a) *enteric fever*, which is the syndrome usually found in infections by *S. typhi* and *S. paratyphi*, but is also occasionally caused by other serovars; and (b) *salmonella enteritis*, the syndrome usually referred to as *salmonella food poisoning*.

4.2.1 Typhoid and paratyphoid fevers

Typhoid fever in particular has been classically associated with contaminated water as the primary means of transmission. However, as a country develops a more reliable nationwide distribution of treated drinking water, food becomes the more common method of transmission. Because of the restricted natural host range, a human carrier will always be involved in causing an outbreak of typhoid fever or of paratyphoid A fever.

4.2.2 Salmonella enteritis

This is often called gastro enteritis, but in fact there is no gastritis, so it is more accurate to use the term 'enteritis'. In salmonella enteritis, the organisms multiply in the intestinal lumen with diarrhoea being evident after an incubation period of 12–24 hours from the time of consumption of the food. This type of infection can lead to severe dehydration, collapse and death, although salmonella food poisoning is normally a non-fatal self-limiting infection in healthy adults. *Salmonella* can however cause septicaemia in about 1 % of cases, and with some serovars the rate for systemic infection may be much higher; for example, in the UK *S. dublin* enteritis may have a 3–5 % incidence of septicaemia, and *S. virchow* enteritis may show a 6 % incidence.

In a given country, there may be a long-established involvement of specific food products, but at any time a new food vehicle may become involved, or a new serovar may appear. The involvement may be of short duration, if it has been brought about by, for example, a failure in hygiene or in Good Manufacturing Practice (GMP) in a factory. In this case, after an identification of the source by epidemiological investigation, appropriate measures may eliminate this particular risk. In recent years in the UK for example, we have seen outbreaks caused by *S. napoli* in imported chocolate, *S. ealing* in infant feeds, *S. saintpaul* and *S. virchow* in mung bean sprouts, and *S. typhimurium* in a vacuum-packed 'shelf-stable' salami-type snack food. In all these cases, the incidence of the organisms in hazardous numbers was caused by a lack of hygiene or failure to observe GMP at the premises producing the foods. In the case of the *S. napoli* outbreak, public health microbiologists were able to ascertain that enteritis could follow consumption of as few as six to 10 organisms.

A new vehicle or the appearance of a serovar new to the country may cause a substantial and long-term shift in the relative significances of either serovars or food vehicles or both. For example, *S. agona* and *S. hadar* were introduced into the UK poultry flock in the 1960s and 1970s respectively by imported contaminated animal feed constituents. Although now reduced in significance they must now be regarded as part of the normal UK microflora, but they do not seem to have altered the nature of the hazard presented by poultry or hen eggs. The recent build-up of *S. enteritidis* PT4 in poultry in the UK and other European countries has had a somewhat different level of significance. This phage type causes a high rate of systemic infection in chickens, and there is a significant rate of transovarian spread which leads to vertical transmission:

Infected adult → egg → embryo → chick → infected adult

In addition, the egg becomes a significant possible source of infection in human beings. Furthermore, *S. enteritidis* PT4 causes the slow development of a pericardial lesion containing vast numbers of bacteria in the infected chicken. When the pericardial sac is burst by a mechanical eviscerator in a poultry processing plant, the processing line will then contaminate at least the next 100 carcasses.

The rise in human enteritis caused by *S. enteritidis* PT4 has resulted in a range of new or revised government legislation. For example, in the UK, there have been the Zoonoses Order 1989, the Testing of Poultry Flocks Order 1989, and a new Protein Processing Order. It is necessary for the food-retailing industry to alter its practices. Eggs should be distributed and retailed under the protection of a complete 'cold chain'. Without this protection, any salmonellae present may multiply extensively. Obviously, for the same reason, the consumer needs to store eggs under refrigeration, and to recognize that eggs so stored must receive more thorough heating to reach the same temperature than eggs kept at ambient temperature. Advice to the industry and to the consumer has remained inadequate and misleading in this regard.

4.3 *Listeria monocytogenes*

Listeria monocytogenes was identified as a potential human pathogen about 60 years ago. Since then, occasional sporadic cases of human listeriosis have been detected, but it is only relatively recently that food has been identified as a possible vehicle of infection. Surveillance of human listeriosis in the UK has been largely passive and laboratory-based, and for a long period there were between 20 and 50 cases per annum. In the last decade, there has been an increase in confirmed listeriosis to around 300 cases per annum. The high case fatality rate (30–50 % of identified cases) has ensured that positive identifications would not go unnoticed.

There are however, a number of problems to be solved in the aetiology of listeriosis:

1. The bacterium is very widely distributed and common in natural environments but the disease is rare.

2. A small but significant proportion of the human population may be carrying the bacterium asymptomatically at any one time (e.g. in Denmark one study suggested 1 % of the population).

3. There are no reliable data on the minimum infective dose.

4. The susceptibility to clinical listeriosis is much greater in certain sectors of the population, especially pregnant women and their foetuses, neonates, immunodeficient and immunocompromised people. Late-onset disease in neonates often derives from cross-infection within a maternity hospital.

5. The incubation period in adult disease can be up to several weeks.

Selective enrichment and isolation procedures for the organism were improved substantially in the 1970s, and as a result of a number of well-documented foodborne outbreaks in the 1970s and 1980s, foods are increasingly being monitored for the presence of *L. monocytogenes*. Since the organism is ubiquitous (it occurs in water, soil, and on plant materials) and psychrotrophic, it is not surprising that it is found in many foods. What is worrying are the high counts that are sometimes found.

It has been reported that growth on food at refrigeration temperatures is accompanied by an induction of listeriolysin production. Although this compound does not seem to be responsible for any of the clinical manifestations, it appears to have a rôle in the entrance of the organism into the body tissues.

Listeria monocytogenes is somewhat heat resistant for a vegetative bacterium; for example one study found that in ice cream the D value at 68.3°C was 231 seconds, and at 73.9°C was 31 seconds.

There have been a number of simultaneous developments in the food industries in developed countries, especially in relation to ready-prepared meals which have tended to favour an increase in the presence and numbers of *L. monocytogenes* in food at the time of consumption:

1. A great increase in the sale of cook–chill products. These may receive inadequate initial cooking and/or may also suffer post-cooking contamination.

2. Refrigeration seems to help resuscitation of any heat-damaged bacteria, and also induces listeriolysin production and thus increases virulence.

3. Products with extended refrigerated shelf-lives are being expected by both catering establishments (e.g. hospitals) and the domestic consumer.

4. Reheating of cook–chill foods is often inefficiently carried out in microwave ovens. In one survey it was found that *Listeria* survived in 22 of 27 (81 %) contaminated food items reheated in microwave ovens according to the oven manufacturers' instructions.

4.4 *Escherichia coli* and *Shigella*

The food industry has had some difficulty in coming to terms with the possibility of *Escherichia coli* being an enteric pathogen rather than a normally harmless intestinal commensal organism which on occasions can become an opportunistic pathogen when transferred to other sites in the body. Many food microbiologists therefore continue to regard the presence of *E. coli* in terms of its *indicator* or *index* status. In fact, *E. coli* and *Shigella* are not distinguishable by DNA : DNA hybridization, and today it is felt that the differences between *Escherichia* and *Shigella* do not support separate generic status. One of the problems is that only certain serovars do have enteric pathogenic capability, and in the past the serotyping of all isolates of *E. coli* would have been an unacceptable financial burden. However, new rapid methods of detecting particular serovars will bring the possibility of monitoring foods for the presence of the pathogenic serovars, and of separating this activity from detecting and counting coliforms, etc. as index or indicator organisms.

Four groups are currently recognized in respect of pathogenicity.

4.4.1 Enterotoxigenic E. coli *(ETEC)*

These include serovars such as O6, O8, O15, O25, O27, O63, and O78. They are relatively rare in temperate climate countries and in areas of good hygiene and good nutrition. However, in the UK they caused a number of hospital outbreaks in the 1970s and 1980s. They are a major cause of infantile enteritis and mortality in tropical countries. Two types of toxin are produced, LT (heat-labile) and ST (heat-stable). In one study of 240 isolates of *E. coli* from foods in the UK, 19 isolates were toxigenic and eight of these produced both toxins. In addition to the enterotoxins, ETEC also needs to possess fimbriae ('CF antigen' – CFA) in order to colonize the gut; CFA-negative strains do not cause diarrhoea.

4.4.2 Enteropathogenic E. coli *(EPEC)*

Serovars such as O26, O55, O86, and O111 fall into this category. Many strains have been shown to have an adhesion mechanism, associated with a plasmid, which enables them to adhere to the brush-border villi of the intestinal epithelium. This adhesion phenomenon can be demonstrated in tissue culture. These organisms can be involved particularly in hospital outbreaks of infantile enteritis that may have a high case fatality rate.

4.4.3 Verocytotoxic E. coli *(VTEC)*

The strains that are verocytotoxic are predominantly of serological group O157, but verocytotoxic strains of other serological groups have been described including of O26 and O128. This category of pathogenicity is defined on the basis of cytotoxicity being demonstrated in tissue cultures of the Vero cell line from the kidney of the African green monkey. The organisms are capable of causing haemorrhagic colitis and haemolytic uraemia syndrome. The probable principal means of transmission is by food. However, one of the major problems is that the minimum infective dose is very low – around 10–100 organisms – and selective enrichment procedures to detect small numbers in foods have been rather inadequate. In 1985–86, 31 % of cases of haemorrhagic colitis in England and Wales were caused by VTEC, mostly one serovar, O157 (and especially O157:H7), being responsible. (See also PHLS 1990a, b.)

Table 4.1 Phenotypic responses of EIEC and *Shigella*

Character	% positive	
	EIEC	*Shigella*
Motility	26	0 (by definition)
Gas from glucose	58	2
Lactose fermentation	49	12
Lysine decarboxylase	17	0 (by definition)

4.4.4 *Enteroinvasive* E. coli *(EIEC)*

DNA–DNA hybridization experiments show there to be essentially a taxonomic concordance of EIEC with *Shigella*, and there is considerable serological relatedness, with the two types of organism being differentiated primarily by phenotypic responses as shown in Table 4.1.

The following are equivalent: *E. coli* O124 and *S. dysenteriae* 3; *E. coli* O143 and *S. boydii* 8; *E. coli* O152 and *S. dysenteriae* 12. However, at present, both nomenclatural designations are still used. As far as is known these organisms naturally infect only human beings, there being no other known animal reservoir.

In a survey in Thailand in 1985, 4 % of children with diarrhoea were found to be infected with EIEC. In England and Wales, more than 75 % of isolations of EIEC and *Shigella* are of *S. sonnei*; the number of isolations has dropped from *c*. 45 000 per annum in the 1950s to *c*. 5000 in 1989.

4.5 *Yersinia enterocolitica*

Yersinia enterocolitica was first recognized in 1964. It is psychrotrophic, growing well at 4°C and capable of growth down to 0°C. Selective isolation can be based on incubation of fairly typical *Enterobacteriaceae* isolation media (e.g. MacConkey's agar or S.S. agar) at 4°C.

Of the 34 serovars, serovars 3 and 9 are most commonly involved in enteritis in Europe. In northern Europe, *Y. enterocolitica* isolations from patients with enteritis can be equivalent to about 20 % of the number of *Salmonella* isolations. The infection is characterized by diarrhoea, fever and abdominal pain, especially in young children. It is easily misdiagnosed as appendicitis. Septicaemia can occur, especially in the old, leading to various complications such as arthritis or meningitis.

The organism has been isolated from milk, ice cream, meat (particularly pork), and seafoods.

4.6 *Vibrio parahaemolyticus*

Vibrio parahaemolyticus is a moderate halophile of marine origin, that inhabits coastal and estuarine waters in warm temperate and sub-tropical regions. It shows a seasonal cycle related to water temperature, overwintering in the marine sediments. After consuming a food containing the organisms, there is an incubation period of 12–24 hours, followed by diarrhoea with associated severe abdominal pain. The infection is usually self-limiting, lasting a few days, although fatalities have been recorded. Obviously, the foods particularly associated with this food poisoning are seafoods, and particularly shellfish and crustacea taken from estuarine and coastal waters. Since the bacterium is heat-sensitive, either the food will have been consumed raw, or a cooked food will have been cross-contaminated after cooking. Many countries apply a Microbiological Guideline or Microbiological Specification to imported shellfish and crustacea in relation to this organism.

4.7 *Vibrio cholerae*

Vibrio cholerae is known mainly as the cause of waterborne epidemics of cholera, an explosive diarrhoea that kills 40 % or more of infected untreated individuals. Foodborne infections can be caused by shellfish or salad vegetables (in neither case does multiplication in the vehicle appear necessary). However, *V. cholerae* is capable of extensive growth on a variety of foods and so it seems likely that in some cases cholera occurs as an infection-type food poisoning.

Treatment is now generally by oral rehydration therapy – the drinking of sugar and sodium chloride in water, which replaces the water lost by diarrhoea.

Several other species of the genus *Vibrio* cause intestinal diseases that are of various degrees of severity; many of the cases are associated with the consumption of infected food, often shellfish.

4.8 *Aeromonas*

Aeromonas bacteria have long been known to be common contaminants of low-acid foods of high a_w, and to be capable of growth on such foods at ambient and refrigerator temperatures. Recently several reports have appeared of diarrhoea, particularly in young children, in which *Aeromonas* was the sole agent incriminated. These bacteria have several features (e.g. production of cytotoxin and haemolysin, adherence to intestinal wall) considered to be characteristic of enteric pathogens, but there is not yet a clear indication of the importance of *Aeromonas* as a cause of infection-type food poisoning.

4.9 *Clostridium perfringens*

Food poisoning caused by *Clostridium perfringens* was first described in 1895, although modern epidemiological studies date from 1945. Although it can be quite common, especially in the context of mass catering of meat dishes such as stews, casseroles, and reheated, sliced roast meats, in recent years the disease has been overshadowed by others of greater clinical hazard.

Food poisoning principally involves Type A strains, as the result of ingestion of large numbers of viable organisms, which then produce an enterotoxin as they sporulate in the gut, causing abdominal pain and diarrhoea lasting for about 12 hours. In Britain a typical aetiology is the preparation, cooking and cooling of large bulks of meat dishes, permitting the survival, heat activation and subsequent germination of the spores, to give counts of vegetative cells in the food as high as 10^7 or even 10^8 per gram.

Rarely, *C. perfringens* Type C may cause a much more serious and even fatal disease known as enteritis necroticans, in which there is damage to jejunum, ileum and colon. Outbreaks of this have been described in Germany, and also in Papua New Guinea; in the latter case it is associated with eating of pigs at ceremonial feasts, and is called pigbel.

5
Organoleptic spoilage of food by microorganisms

5.1 What is food spoilage?

Food spoilage is a change in food making it unsafe, less acceptable or unacceptable to the consumer for its original purpose. Thus, food may be spoiled by being contaminated with disease-causing organisms that may not be organoleptically detected by the consumer, by contamination with glass, pieces of metal or paint, by undergoing chemical change (e.g. rancidity), or by the growth of microorganisms that may become manifest in a variety of ways. Such a definition excludes: foods that are inherently dangerous, such as insufficiently boiled red kidney beans; foods that are inherently poor because of lack of flavour resulting from poor choice of raw materials or recipes; foods that are inherently dangerous to certain allergic individuals; and foods that may cause illness through excessive consumption. The definition includes assessment by the consumer; in other words it allows for a certain subjectivity, and it recognizes that change may occur to produce another food, for example cream to sour cream, which nonetheless is 'spoilage' unless the change was deliberately intended. Chapters 3 and 4 have dealt with the ways in which the growth of microorganisms can spoil food by rendering it unsafe. This chapter considers the ways in which organoleptic spoilage due to microorganisms may occur. Various preservation procedures that have been developed to stop, or retard, microbial growth on food are considered in Chapters 6 and 7.

5.2 How microbial spoilage of food occurs

Microbial spoilage of food occurs only if the food is of a type that will support growth of the contaminating microorganisms, *and* such microorganisms have gained access to the food at some stage, *and* the food, once contaminated, is kept for long enough under conditions suitable for enough multiplication to occur to make it unacceptable to the consumer. Factors involved have been discussed by Mossel & Ingram (1955; see Section 16.3).

5.3 The ability of a food to support microbial growth

Microorganisms require adequate nutrients, suitable gaseous conditions, appropriate temperature and pH value, sufficient available water, and absence of inhibitors in order to be able to grow (Chapter 1). If any one of these items is not within the required range there will be no growth. Some foods naturally contain specific antimicrobial substances. For example, bovine milk contains lactoferrin and the lactoperoxidase system; egg white contains lysozyme, and iron-binding conalbumin, which retards growth by withholding iron; and various plants contain essential oils, tannins or anthocyanins with microbistatic or microbicidal properties.

It is clear from Chapter 1 that there are many types of microorganisms with respect to growth requirements, and so it follows that a food that is unsatisfactory for the growth of one type of microorganism may be very satisfactory for the growth of another. For example, a food that has been partially dried may have insufficient available water (Section 6.5) to support the growth of most bacteria but may have sufficient to support moulds. Moulds may therefore be able to flourish on such a food because bacterial competition will have been reduced or eliminated. Orange juice is sufficiently acidic to inhibit the growth of many bacteria, although lactic acid bacteria may be part of the spoilage flora because they flourish in acidic conditions. However, they will be able to grow only if yeast have first established themselves, because the bacteria require growth factors, not inherently present in the orange juice, that are provided by the yeast cells. The experience of an animal shortly before slaughter markedly affects the quality of meat produced. If the animal is rested before slaughter glycogen is present in the muscle tissue and so, after slaughter, when oxygen is no longer supplied by

the blood, anaerobic metabolism occurs in the muscle at the expense
of the glycogen to produce lactic acid, which lowers the pH value of
the meat. However, if the animal is stressed, muscle glycogen will be
depleted before death so that after slaughter the pH value of the meat
does not fall. Such a difference in pre-slaughter conditions can result
in a pH difference between 5.5 and 6.5, the higher pH value meat
developing a distinct character – a dark appearance and firm and dry
to the touch (so-called DFD meat) – and spoiling much more quickly.
Foods such as uncut vegetables and fruit will be partly protected from
microbial spoilage by their skin which, besides providing a barrier to
entry, will have a low a_w; removal or puncture of the skin, or slicing
may expose relatively unprotected, high a_w layers which may readily
support growth. For a bacterium or fungus to succeed as a pathogen
on the living plant, or as a primary saprophyte on the plant material
immediately after harvest or slaughter, in the absence of mechanical
damage it will need to have developed enzyme systems capable of
breaking down these barriers. For example, pectinases will facilitate
spread through a plant tissue and cellulases will breach the plant cell
walls and make the plant cytoplasm available to the microorganisms
outside the plant cells. Once these mechanical barriers have been broken
down, other microorganisms not possessing such enzymes may then
play an important part in spoilage.

In theory at least, microorganisms may be prevented from growing
by the absence of one key nutrient, but in practice a relatively small
amount may be sufficient for spoilage to occur.

5.4 Sources of microbial contamination of food

It should be assumed that all potential spoilage microorganisms are
everywhere and that if a food is capable of supporting microbial growth,
and is kept for long enough under conditions that will allow
contamination and growth, then spoilage will occur. Obviously there
will be a microflora associated with the raw material as a natural habitat,
such as yeasts on fruit, staphylococci on the epidermes of mammals,
pseudomonads and alteromonads on the skin of fish, corynebacteria in
bovine milk, and so on. Descriptions of the natural microflorae of raw
materials can be found in various texts (e.g. Harrigan & McCance,
1976; ICMSF, 1980). Nevertheless, there are many circumstances that
can lead to an increased amount of contamination and hence more

rapid spoilage. Contamination of the material may be caused by microorganisms coming from air, soil, water, faeces, etc. Airborne contamination can often provide an important source of mould spores (especially from those microfungi that produce the very light spores such as conidia which are intended for airborne dispersal). Having windows of a factory open, with wind blowing in contamination from refuse containers situated elsewhere on the factory premises, can markedly increase the risk of mould spoilage of products, as can failure to remove crumbs from a cooling area for pork pies – the pies undergoing mould spoilage by, as they cool, taking in spores produced by mould growing on old crumbs. Sometimes air can be a source of the more resistant bacterial forms (especially spores of the endospore-forming bacteria); for example, *Bacillus* spores may contaminate milk by airborne distribution from dry, dusty animal feeds (e.g. hay) if the cattle are fed at the same time as being milked.

Careless evisceration of animals in the slaughterhouse may increase the contamination of the carcass with gut microorganisms, thus increasing the risk both of rapid spoilage and carriage of salmonellae and other food-poisoning organisms. The use of large tanks for communal washing of chicken carcasses can spread such contamination between carcasses, although the extent of this will depend on the relative flow of carcasses and water through the tank, as well as on chlorine concentration in the water. Fat rendered from waste material at a slaughterhouse and loaded into uncleaned drums may become contaminated by mould that has grown on a protective layer of grease on the drum inner surface so that, if kept at tropical temperature, emulsions may break down to produce areas of sufficiently high a_w, the fat becoming mouldy. Dried onion, as may be used in poultry stuffing, may carry a heavy load of spores of *Clostridium perfringens*, so providing an inoculum that can result in the poultry causing *C. perfringens* food poisoning. Soil brought into the factory or kitchen on raw vegetables is another source of this organism. Inadequate cleaning of food containers after use results in the accumulation of a flora that can then contaminate fresh food placed in the re-used containers. In this way, heavy inoculations of spoilage organisms can occur, for example from fish boxes on to raw fish or from milk-holding tanks into milk. Handling of cooked food after raw food, without washing hands and utensils, provides many opportunities for recontamination of the cooked food. Absence of a sense of personal hygiene by food handlers affords many opportunities for contamination: scratching of

spots; not covering infected cuts; not washing hands after using the
toilet or after handling contaminated material or pets; spitting or
sneezing into the food. Allowing access of rats, mice, birds, flies, cats
and dogs to stored food increases the risk of microbial contamination,
these sources being thought of as particularly important in the context
of introduction of enteric bacteria.

5.5 Types of organoleptic spoilage of foods

If foods can support the growth of microorganisms and contamination
occurs, then storage under conditions that allow growth may cause the
food to become unacceptable for a variety of microbiological reasons.
Microorganisms may produce compounds with offensive odours, for
example amines and sulphides from meat or trimethylamine from
marine fish. They may alter the appearance of the food by colouring
or discolouring it, or by becoming visible as slime or as a fluffy
mycelium. They may produce a textural change, such as the liquefaction
of vegetables by means of pectinolytic enzymes, or the development of
ropiness in milk. Microorganisms may also produce changes in flavour,
more usually by adding a component to the food but sometimes by
removing a flavour component by metabolizing it.

Procedures for preservation involve either altering the nature of the
food or its storage so as to stop or retard growth (Chapter 6), or killing
some or all of the microorganisms in the food (Chapter 7). Such
procedures, unless all microorganisms are totally inactivated, usually
lead to a different type of spoilage, albeit delayed, from that which
would have occurred with the unprocessed food. The environment will
have been changed, so favouring a different type of microbial
community. For example, in the production of milk and dairy products
under a traditional agricultural system, with milk being collected into
churns and not subject to refrigerated storage, the acidogenic lactic
acid bacteria are a principal source of spoilage, with the milk souring.
The traditional response in the farm or domestic kitchen to milk
'spoiled' in this way would be to divert it into producing fermented
products such as curd cheese. With the introduction of refrigerated
bulk-tank storage on the farm and transport of the refrigerated milk in
refrigerated tankers to the dairy products factory, lactic acid bacteria
become unimportant, and the spoilage problem is from proteolytic or
lipolytic psychrotrophs. Enzymes from such organisms may persist

after UHT treatment or after cheese manufacture and continue to act on the food material. In some countries that have established a technologically-based food industry in conjunction with the retention of traditional small-farm agriculture, both types of microorganisms may be important. A farmer owning one or a few cows may use churns, and may lack adequate refrigeration equipment – there will thus be some development of lactic acid bacteria in the early stages. If then these churns are delivered by cart to local milk collection centres where the milk is stored in refrigerated bulk tanks before collection and delivery by refrigerated tankers to regional dairy factories, there may be subsequent spoilage by psychrotrophs.

Raw meat packaged in an atmosphere high in carbon dioxide spoils more readily from *Brochothrix* than from pseudomonads and other Gram-negative bacteria. Dried meat or fish, if drying is not sufficient to stop all microbial growth, will spoil by moulds or yeasts, whereas the undried product would have been spoiled by bacteria.

There are many such examples of changes in foods and implications for changing microbial spoilage and hazards of which the food scientist must be aware. Reference should be made to the texts in the bibliography for more details of this subject.

The essential point is that organoleptic spoilage of food by microorganisms is an important problem and can take many forms. The procedures involving hygiene and preservation for controlling microbial food poisoning discussed in this book are in most cases equally applicable to the control of organoleptic spoilage.

6
Procedures designed to stop microbial growth in food

6.1 The need to understand

If a raw or processed food is to be wholesome and safe for the consumer it will usually have had to be subjected to one or more processes and storage procedures chosen, hopefully at least in part, to minimize risk of disease and to stop or retard spoilage. Some of these processes and procedures have been developed over thousands of years; others are relatively new. They all require to be understood by the modern food processor so that their limitations and risks can be appreciated. This is particularly important now that several techniques may be used in combination. Their application is becoming more sophisticated as workers develop predictive modelling procedures to facilitate choice of the best combinations of conditions for stopping the development of microbiological problems in foods. This chapter and Chapter 7 will consider aspects of various preservation and processing procedures as a basis for understanding the types of control and monitoring that such procedures may require. In this chapter we will concentrate on processes that are aimed primarily at retarding or suspending growth rather than at killing organisms. It is important to realize that foods exposed to such processes can be at least as dangerous or perishable as the raw foods once they are removed from conditions imposed by the process. Furthermore, inhibitory conditions may actually favour the growth of a pathogen (e.g. *Listeria* at refrigerator temperatures) by inhibiting its natural competitors.

6.2 The relevance of the lag phase and of exponential change

Cleanliness of raw materials, machinery and staff all play an important part in the quality of a processed or preserved food partly because many preservation methods act by retarding growth rather than by killing microbes or completely stopping growth. Control is achieved at two stages: at the lag phase, the phase before increase in numbers begins, which can be made to last for longer; and during the log or exponential phase, when the growth rate is reduced (i.e. the time taken for the population to double – the *doubling time* or *mean generation time* – is increased). Heavy contamination may affect one or both of these phases. The lag phase is often shorter when the contaminating population is large, because the organisms can more rapidly establish optimum conditions of oxidation–reduction potential, CO_2 concentration, etc. The growth *rate* is not generally affected by numbers, but the *number* of microbes produced in a given time will depend on the number present on the food at the start of the time. Thus, if a contaminant bacterium has a generation time of 4 hours at 5°C, and there are 100 g^{-1} present, a day after the end of the lag phase there will still be only 6400 g^{-1} present. If, however, there are $10\,000 \text{ g}^{-1}$ present initially, the number after 24 hours will be $640\,000 \text{ g}^{-1}$. The generation time is the same in both cases, but $623\,700 \text{ g}^{-1}$ *more* bacteria will have been produced during the same period in the latter case than in the former. Cleanliness of products to be exposed to a treatment designed to kill contaminating organisms is also important because death rate is often exponential, rather than all the organisms dying together. Under these circumstances the larger the initial population of contaminants, the longer will be the treatment time required to achieve the same probability of sterility.

6.3 Refrigeration

6.3.1 The use of refrigerators

Refrigeration is usually defined as the process of storing items at temperatures between -1 and $+8$°C without the item undergoing any physically induced change such as the production of ice crystals. However some foods, particularly some fruits and starchy materials, may be damaged by storage at refrigeration temperatures. Beef and mutton can become tough if they are stored below 10°C within 10 hours of slaughter unless special techniques are used. It is becoming increasingly recognized that the upper end of the refrigeration temperature range should not be used for products that rely entirely on low temperature to prevent the growth of food-poisoning organisms, but only for foods such as yoghurt, fermented meats and hard cheeses, in which additional preservation factors are operating. Storage under refrigeration retards deterioration, but the life of a food that is rapidly perishable at room temperature will not be greatly extended by this procedure. It is the responsibility of manufacturers to determine the shelf life of chilled foods and to use this information to set the expiry date indicated on the product label.

The refrigerator should be big enough for the amount of use, so that there is sufficient space for cold air to circulate, and the refrigeration unit should be powerful enough to maintain the required temperature under all conditions of use. A firm distinction should be recognized between units with refrigeration power sufficient only to *maintain* the temperature of an already chilled food and those which are able to *reduce* the temperature to the storage temperature as well as to maintain it once achieved. Manufacturers of chilled foods such as airline meals must ensure, by careful use of probes in samples of products in the form and in the bulk containers in which they are dispatched, that the temperature of the products is reduced to the required level. Failure to attend to this detail leads to products spending insufficient time in chiller rooms so that they are dispatched warm, allowing unacceptable amounts of microbial growth to occur. Raw foods such as raw meat, which can be expected to carry food-poisoning and food-spoilage organisms, must not be stored with processed food which is to be eaten without further cooking, nor should staff handle cooked foods after raw foods without first washing, and preferably changing overalls, to avoid cross-contamination.

6.3.2 Effects of refrigeration on microorganisms in food

Reduction in temperature below the optimum for microbes causes an increase in the generation time and changes in the composition of the cells. The generation time of a pseudomonad might be 1 hour at 20°C, 2.5 hours at 10°C, 5 hours at 5°C, 8 hours at 2°C and 11 hours at 0°C. At 5°C or less most mesophilic microbes do not grow, and may die, possibly because destructive processes in the cell cannot be countered sufficiently quickly by repair metabolism. However the situation is more complex than this because some organisms incapable of growth at low temperatures, for example campylobacters, or incapable of growth on the food at all, for example viruses, appear to survive better in refrigerators than at room temperature, presumably because the growth of other organisms that damage them is retarded or inhibited and/or because lethal denaturation reactions are retarded. Even if the growth of organisms is stopped it does not necessarily mean that all metabolism associated with them will cease. Thus, preformed microbial enzymes may continue functioning and so damage food at temperatures below that at which the organism is able to grow. However, because the rate of all chemical and biochemical reactions is reduced by lowering the temperature, the greatest preservative effect of refrigeration is achieved by the use of as low a temperature as possible.

Storage at refrigerator temperatures has a marked effect on the type of spoilage or other changes that eventually occurs, compared with that which would occur at room temperature. The quality of surface-ripened cheeses such as Limburger can be markedly affected, even within the refrigerator range, because minor changes in temperature will alter the balance of activities of the microbial community involved. Raw milk stored at temperatures close to 0°C tends to putrefy because of activity of pseudomonads, rather than to sour due to activity of lactic acid bacteria. *Listeria* and *Yersinia* may be favoured over many other organisms because they are capable of growth at 4°C whereas many of the organisms that compete with them at ambient temperatures are not. Thus, *ignoring other risks*, risk of listeriosis or yersiniosis in consumers may actually be increased by refrigeration of foods as compared with storage at ambient temperature.

Both growth and survival of microbes at refrigerator temperatures will be affected by the nature of the food, a principle which is used in devising appropriate combined processes (Section 7.6).

6.4 Freezing

Freezing of foods is usually taken to mean the establishment and maintenance of a temperature that is sufficiently below 0°C to stop microbial growth and to at least severely retard any chemical changes and activities of enzymes. In practice this means the establishment of a temperature of around $-18°C$ and maintenance at that temperature throughout the distribution chain, with attention to such details as rapid transfer to freezers from vans on delivery to retail outlets and ensuring that chest freezer displays are not over-filled.

It is the removal from the system of available water by the formation of ice crystals that is responsible for the cessation of microbial growth. In fact, organisms capable of growing at sub-zero temperatures are also capable of growing at low a_w values (Section 6.5). Many food organisms are killed by the process of freezing, the greatest death occurring if freezing is slow and the temperature is only a little below $0°C$ – conditions which have to be avoided because they also cause maximum damage to food being frozen. Some microbes will also die as a result of storage at the freezer temperature. Nevertheless, if a food were contaminated before freezing, many microbes will remain alive, so one must recognize that some frozen foods (e.g. raw poultry), either in the frozen state or when thawed, may be the source of microbes to contaminate other foods. Thawed frozen foods may be more liable to spoilage and to be the source of more food-poisoning organisms than the fresh counterparts. The freezing process will have damaged the food, so that on thawing nutrients for contaminating microbes are released from damaged cells of the food, and entry of microbes beneath the surface of the food is facilitated. The dripping of fluids, that may contain many microbes, from thawed frozen foods on to work surfaces and other foods can add to the potential risk. When examining frozen foods for the presence of microbes it is important to realize that some organisms may be damaged so that they cannot be recovered using normal selective isolation procedures unless they have first been put through a resuscitation stage to allow repair of the injury. Many examples of this phenomenon are being discovered and modifications to isolation procedures for specific organisms are being made, so we must treat some old reports of the inability of organisms to survive freezing with caution. It may be that the organisms *were* alive at the time of sampling but died when exposed to the harsh selective media and incubation conditions used.

6.5 Drying, sugar and salt – the reduction of water activity

All microbes require water for their growth because water is their major constituent and because it is used in many metabolic reactions and in the transport of susbtances into and out of them. Thus, removal of water from a food will stop microbial growth and so serve as a preservation process. It is not necessary to remove *all* the water from the food. The same effect can be achieved by the addition of solutes without actually *removing* any water at all, and a similar effect is achieved by freezing, when the water remains but is unavailable because it is locked in ice crystals.

To understand the control of microbial growth in this way we have to consider the concept of water activity (a_w). The following simplification may prove helpful. Water molecules do not have the same electrical state over the whole surface – the oxygen atom tends to be negatively charged and the hydrogen atoms tend to be positively charged. Thus, water molecules tend to be held loosely to each other by hydrogen bonding – the attraction between the negative charge on the oxygen of one molecule and the positive charge on the hydrogen of another molecule. These attractive forces are overcome periodically as a molecule with greater than average energy escapes from the mass of liquid water, giving rise to vapour pressure. On the other hand the attractive forces become more important when the temperature is lowered sufficiently that movement of molecules is reduced to allow the formation of an extensive crystalline structure (freezing). Microbes 'draw' water molecules into themselves from these loose associations in liquid water. When solutes are added the relationships of the water molecules in liquid water change. They tend to be drawn around the molecules or ions of the solute, a feature that has several repercussions. Water molecules require greater energy than before to escape into the vapour phase – hence the boiling point of the liquid is raised and the vapour pressure is lowered. They need less energy to escape from the tendency to combine with others in a rigid crystalline structure – hence the freezing point of the liquid is depressed. And it is less easy for microbes to capture water because the molecules are being held as 'clouds' around the solute. Thus, in order to assess the extent to which water in a particular food will be available for microbes one has to assess the extent of the forces tending to restrict movement of the water molecules. This is usually achieved by using one of several methods for measuring the vapour pressure of the food, and is expressed as the a_w where

a_w = vapour pressure of the food/vapour pressure of pure water.

This value usually enables one to predict whether or not microbes will grow in the food, whereas knowing the percentage of water in the food does not, but in a heterogeneous food a low overall a_w value obtained from measuring the vapour pressure above the whole food may mask parts of high a_w which will support growth.

The a_w of most fresh foods is above 0.99. Generally speaking, bacteria are the most sensitive to reduction in water activity (minimum a_w for growth around 0.9), yeasts are less sensitive (minimum a_w 0.88), and moulds are the least sensitive (minimum a_w 0.80), though in all groups there are wide variations. The minimal a_w for any microbial growth is 0.60. Lowering of the a_w below the optimum causes an increase in the lag phase, a reduction in the growth rate, and sometimes an increase in the nutritional requirements of the microbes, these effects being influenced by other factors in the food such as temperature, pH value and presence of inhibitors. Particular aspects of the metabolism of organisms may be specifically affected by reductions in a_w; for example the production of toxins may be inhibited although the organism can continue to grow. Organisms may be damaged by reduction of a_w and so require careful resuscitation for their detection, and some will be killed. One must regard reconstituted dried food as at least as likely to spoil as the original undried food. Many problems that arise with reconstituted dried food being the source of food poisoning or foodborne disease are due to the use of contaminated water and utensils at the time of reconstitution.

6.6 Intermediate moisture foods (IMF)

Foods with an a_w above 0.6 and below 0.85, that is foods which have an a_w sufficient to allow some growth of some moulds and yeasts but not of food-poisoning or of most food-spoilage bacteria, are shelf stable at ambient temperatures for considerable periods. Humectants (added as solutes to reduce a_w without markedly changing the acceptability of the product) and chemical preservatives may be added. The main potential threats to health from IMF are *Staphylococcus aureus*, which has been reported to grow as low as a_w 0.83 (although enterotoxin production is not thought to occur below a_w of 0.86) and moulds, which might produce mycotoxins.

6.7 Changing the gas phase

From the realization that most of the spoilage organisms of high a_w foods stored at refrigerator temperatures are obligate aerobes has come the idea of packing such foods in the absence of oxygen, either as vacuum packs, in which removal of all gases so far as is possible is achieved, or gas packs, in which air is replaced with some other gas, usually nitrogen. In such cases care has to be taken in the choice of wrapping material because several plastics are highly permeable to oxygen. By using vacuum packs or gas packs spoilage is greatly retarded because many of the usual spoilage organisms are unable to grow without oxygen. Similarly, because common spoilage organisms of refrigerated foods are sensitive to high concentrations of CO_2, this gas at concentrations of 10 % has been used in combination with refrigeration, higher concentrations than this leading to the damage of some foods (e.g. 'gas burn' of meat). Great care has to be exercised in the use of these techniques, particularly the removal of oxygen, because they might facilitate the growth of organisms of public-health significance, for example *Clostridium botulinum* and *S. aureus*.

7

Procedures designed to kill microorganisms in food

7.1 Preservation by killing microorganisms

If a food contains no microorganisms, and is protected from future microbiological contamination, it will not be subject to microbiological spoilage or be the source of microbiological disease. This obvious fact has led to the development of several types of processing that involve treating the food in some way to kill all the microbes or at least all those that would be capable of growing in the food and, either before or after this, packaging the food to protect it from subsequent contamination. The most extensively used agent for killing microorganisms is heat. In theory at least, such processes have the advantage that, on completion, the product requires no special storage conditions. The disadvantage is that the killing process, which basically involves inflicting chemical damage on the microbes, will not leave the food unaltered, and so it is necessary to treat the food no more than is needed to achieve a high probability of safety and stability. Such procedures are dependent upon the killing process being reliable, any post-treatment dispensing and packaging being aseptic, and the container remaining unbreached. One must not assume that products prepared in this way will be truly shelf-stable. For example, chemical changes to the product may occur, and containers may corrode.

7.2 Death of microorganisms by heat

There are two classes of microbial states with respect to resistance to the lethal effects of heat. Organisms in the growing state, the so-called vegetative state, will die if the temperature is just a few degrees above the maximum temperature at which growth can occur. For most microorganisms this means that temperatures of 60°C and above are rapidly lethal, although one must not forget the thermophilic bacteria, some of which are capable of growth at temperatures close to 100°C. Some organisms may also exist in a resting state, usually as spores. The spores of most moulds are only marginally more resistant to heat than is the vegetative state, but the endospores produced by *Bacillus* and *Clostridium* bacteria are extremely resistant to heat and dominate consideration of the amount of heat to be applied to a food to render it safe and stable.

The way in which heat causes the death of microbes is not known although there has been much research and many interesting findings. One early view was that a single crucial molecule in each cell has to be damaged for death to occur; another now more accepted view is that heat causes incremental damage and death occurs as a result of a final piece of damage that, taken with all other damage, is lethal. This is known as 'multiple hit target theory' (it could be thought of as a microbiological version of the 'death by a thousand cuts'). However, a simple model (a logarithmic rate of destruction) that enabled the prediction of the efficiency of a heating process in killing a particular type of microorganism in a particular suspending medium was developed many years ago and has found great utility in the food industry. In our discussions we will assume that this model is correct but one must always have in the back of one's mind that it does not fit all the facts and its uncritical application can be misleading in certain regards. Often extremely concave curves (extreme 'tailing') may be seen in a plot of log survivors against time; sometimes, but not always, such data will give a straight line when probit survivors is plotted against log time. Readers interested in the implications of multiple hit target theory for thermal processing are recommended to consult the papers of Moats (1971a, b) and Cerf (1977).

When a suspension of a single type of bacterium in a uniform physiological state (e.g. all vegetative cells in the exponential phase of growth in a batch culture) is held at a lethal temperature the number of viable bacteria is considered to fall logarithmically. Thus, the number dying at a particular time is dependent on the number present. If this were the correct model for thermal death, then a graph of the log of number of survivors (on the y axis) plotted against the time of heating at a particular temperature (plotted on the x axis) should give a straight line, the slope of which indicates the degree of sensitivity of the culture to that particular heating temperature. We can obtain a value, the D value, which indicates this sensitivity of the culture and which is independent of the numbers of organisms involved. The D value is 'the time taken at a particular lethal temperature to kill 90 % of the population', for example from $\log_{10} 4$ to $\log_{10} 3$.

You might consider this further by asking 'How long will it take to achieve the death of *all* the population?'. The answer is that you can *never* be *certain* that all the population has been killed, no matter how long it has been heated. All that is certain is that the longer the culture is heated the greater is the *probability* that all the organisms have been killed. Work this through by imagining that at the start of heating a culture at a particular temperature there were 10 000 live organisms present per millilitre of culture. After heating for four D values there would be one live organism present per millilitre of suspension. After heating for a further D value one could not claim that there was none remaining alive. The population would have been reduced to one live organism per 10 ml, and there would thus be a 1 in 10 chance of there being one live organism present in any 1 ml sampled. After heating for a further D value there would be a 1 in 100 chance of one live organism being present in 1 ml of suspension. No matter how long heating continued one could never predict with certainty that there would be none present. Thus, when deciding on the temperature and time of a heating process, one has to decide on what *probability* of a living organism remaining in the heated product is acceptable.

Heating at a higher temperature kills the organisms more quickly (i.e. the D value will be less). There is a relationship between the rise in temperature and the reduction in D value, which is traditionally shown by plotting the log of D values obtained at different temperatures (on the y axis) against the temperature at which the particular D value was obtained (on the x axis). A straight line is drawn through the points, the steepness of the slope indicating the extent to which raising the temperature increases the killing rate. The slope can be expressed as the z value, which is the temperature coefficient of thermal destruction and is 'the rise in temperature needed to cause a fall of 90 % in the time taken to kill 90 % of the population'.

These two values, the D value and the z value, are of great use in the food industry because they allow one to predict the amount of heating needed to give a certain probability of sterility in a batch of known size. For most canned foods heating times and temperatures are based on the amount of heating needed to reduce an unknown number of endospores of *Clostridium botulinum* to $1/10^{12}$ of that number (i.e. through 12 log cycles), the so-called 12D cook or botulinum cook. In order to compare heating processes with different heating and cooling curves, and to quantify the total lethality of a process, the F value is calculated. The F value of a process is the equivalent time in minutes at 121°C of all the heat received by the product considered with respect to its ability to kill the organism concerned. Heat is not transferred instantaneously throughout a can of food, and so it is necessary to determine what is the overall value of the exposure to high temperature, usually with the 'heating centre' of the can as the reference point. Heat transfer to the centre will be by conduction in a solid food. In a can containing a product with liquid (e.g. canned peas, canned carrots) the heat transfer will be by a combination of convection and conduction (see Stumbo, 1973, for details of the different types of process calculation).

The effectiveness of heat at a particular temperature in killing microorganisms depends not only on the type of organism being heated but also on the nature of the suspending medium. In general, increasing the acidity of the suspending medium decreases D value, while decreasing a_w increases D value. The z value can also be affected by the nature of the suspending medium.

7.2.1 Canning and other heating processes used to achieve a stable product

Heat can be used to inactivate all types of pathogenic and spoilage organisms in canned foods, foods in glass jars and in metal foil and other packs, and foods that are aseptically packed after exposure to heat. The nature of the food with respect to the initial microbial load, the pH value, the water activity (e.g. fat provides 'pockets' of low water activity that may allow organisms to survive), and the viscosity will affect the amount of heat required, as will the size and shape of the container being used. As the most heat-resistant pathogen is *Clostridium botulinum* (as endospores), and as this pathogen causes a severe and often fatal disease, all heating processes of low-acid foods intended to be shelf-stable at ambient temperatures are designed to give a high probability that the organism will not survive. This means that most spoilage organisms are also eliminated, but endospores particularly of the thermophilic *Bacillus* spp. may survive and give rise to spoilage if the containers are stored at high temperatures. Consequently most thermal processes for low-acid foods which would legally require a botulinum cook in fact involve the use of F values substantially greater than the legal minimum. Characteristics of the food may be chosen to reduce the chance of growth of organisms after processing by, for example, the addition of a large amount of sugar as in sweetened condensed milk, nitrite in cured meats, and nisin in strawberries and peas. Certain products of this type, although not acid, may be exempt from a legal requirement for a botulinum cook (e.g. sweetened condensed milk, or catering-pack-sized pasteurized cured hams required to be kept under refrigeration). Foods with a pH value less than 4.6 are widely thought not to present a risk from *C. botulinum* because its endospores usually cannot germinate nor can toxin be produced in such food. For such foods elimination of spoilage organisms, particularly the mould *Byssochlamys fulva*, becomes of greater importance.

7.2.2 Pasteurization

Pasteurization is the name given to a moderate heating process that is intended to kill some types of microbe in a food but not endospores or some other particularly resistant type. Pasteurization may be applied to reduce the risk from pathogens in, for example, milk or to reduce the risk of spoilage of, for example, beer or vinegar. Similar process calculations to those described in Section 7.2 can be performed in respect of a pasteurizing process, although in this case the reference organism is likely to be a non-sporing bacterium or a virus. The pasteurization times for milk (e.g. 63°C for 30 minutes or 72°C for 15 seconds) were chosen because they were sufficient to give a high degree of probability that *Mycobacterium bovis*, one of the most heat-resistant nonsporing pathogens found in milk, would be destroyed. Pasteurized milk has a much longer shelf life than raw milk because most spoilage organisms in the raw milk, particularly lactic acid bacteria and pseudomonads, are also eliminated. When pasteurized milk eventually does spoil the type of spoilage is likely to be completely different from that of raw milk, either because it is brought about by spore formers of the genus *Bacillus* or because of post-pasteurization contamination.

7.2.3 Post-heating contamination

The killing of organisms in a food serves little purpose if access of other organisms to the food is allowed after the heating process. There are several ways in which such access can occur. Assisted cooling of cans after heating is achieved by immersion in water. At this stage a partial vacuum will be created in the can by the cooling of the contents and this may draw water into the can through small temporary faults at the seams. It is therefore necessary to ensure that water used for cooling cans is freed from possible contaminants, usually by chlorination. Also, after immersion, cans should be kept in clean surroundings until they have reached ambient temperature so as to avoid entry of contaminants from other sources in a similar manner. There are advantages to heating products first and packaging them afterwards. Heating can be better controlled, allowing the production of foods with less heat damage (e.g. UHT milk compared with in-bottle sterilized milk) and processing can be continuous. But such procedures make aseptic filling into sterilized packs a crucial stage of the process, a stage that must be carefully monitored. Post-pasteurization contamination of milk is a common occurrence. The finding of nonsporulating bacteria in pasteurized milk or in other heated products always strongly suggests that contamination has occurred after heating.

7.2.4 The lethal effects on microorganisms of cooking

The heating of foods as part of the cooking process may render food safer and give it a longer shelf life than the uncooked food. However, there are many microbiological hazards associated with the cooking of foods, particularly meat. Raw meat should be assumed to have on it a variety of microbes including the pathogens *Salmonella*, *Campylobacter* and *Clostridium perfringens*. Roasting or boiling will kill all bacteria on the surface, excepting some spores. The muscle tissue of a healthy animal at death will usually be virtually sterile and problems will arise only in exceptional circumstances. However, during preparation, rolled or otherwise made up pieces of meat and stuffed poultry may become grossly contaminated with microorganisms such as endospores of *C. perfringens*, which may be protected from heat by the meat. For this reason, large rolled joints and stuffed poultry should be eaten promptly after cooking. Joints of meat or poultry intended to be refrigerated after cooking should be limited in size to that which can be cooled rapidly by the chilling facility available, and then refrigerated so as to avoid germination and growth of *C. perfringens* endospores. Spit roasting of poultry may give a product which looks cooked but which contains, in protected areas like those under the wing, live salmonellae that may grow while the cooling bird is on display. All cooked meats should be kept separate from raw meats to avoid them becoming contaminated with pathogens by cross-contamination.

Microwave cooking is satisfactory if it heats the food to the same temperature and for the same length of time as would be used in a satisfactory traditional cooking procedure. Microwaves have no inherent lethality other than that due to temperature rise resulting from the absorption of the microwaves by water in the food. Some problems may arise, particularly with frozen foods, from the tendency of microwaves to heat some parts while other parts remain cold, even frozen, so protecting pathogens present in these cold parts.

7.3 Irradiation

Like heat, ionizing radiation, from a radioactive substance such as cobalt 60 or from a high-energy electron source, can be used to kill some types (radurization or radicidation – equivalent to pasteurization) or all types (radappertization). The sensitivity of a particular strain of microorganism in a particular suspending medium is indicated by the radiation D value, which is the dose of radiation needed to cause a 90 % reduction in the number of survivors. Efficiency of irradiation is affected by a variety of factors such as temperature, protein content of the suspending medium, water activity, presence of oxygen, etc. The greater the dose of radiation the more extensive is the change in organoleptic quality of the food. One of the anxieties surrounding the introduction of irradiation of foods is that the process may be used to treat food that would otherwise be detectable as unacceptable, in which possibly toxins had already accumulated, for example.

Ultraviolet light is a non-ionizing radiation that is lethal only to microorganisms on surfaces or in clear liquids such as water.

7.4 The use of chemicals

Preservation of foods by the deliberate addition of chemicals (e.g. salts) or by the use of microorganisms to produce chemicals (e.g. lactic acid, acetic acid) has been practised since ancient times. Salting preserves mainly by reducing the a_w, but if nitrites are present (or less commonly, nitrates, from which nitrites can be formed by the activities of some microorganisms), specific lethal effects of the weak acid nitrous acid on the microbes will occur.

Lactic acid, acetic acid, and citric acid also are lethal to many microorganisms. Since these three acids are common constituents of normal and traditional foods, the amounts which may be added are not restricted by legislation. Consequently, although they are weak acids, they are used as acidulants, and have a preservative action by virtue of the low pH value achieved in the food.

Several other weak acids (e.g. benzoic acid; propionic acid; sorbic acid; sulphur dioxide, which in solution gives sulphurous acid) are used as preservatives, but in these cases the amounts and uses are limited by legislation, the small amounts permitted having a negligible effect on the pH value of the food. These inactivate microorganisms only if they are in the form of the undissociated molecule, in which state they are able to enter the microbial cell, release hydrogen ions, and eliminate the proton gradient across the cell membrane, which is crucial to the functioning of the organism. Thus, these agents are most effective at pH values at or below their pK (the pH at which 50 % of the molecules are undissociated). Raising the pH value by one unit will reduce the concentration of undissociated acid by 90 % and so reduce the lethal effect. Thus one must be careful to use such agents at appropriate pH values and to expect changes in pH value to alter their efficiency.

Other chemical inhibitors are used for particular purposes. The non-medical antibiotic, nisin, is added to certain canned products to prevent outgrowth of germinating endospores of spoilage organisms, thereby allowing a lesser heat treatment than would otherwise be necessary to inhibit spoilage. It is also added to certain cheeses to prevent spoilage by clostridia. Ethylene oxide and propylene oxide have been used to fumigate dried fruits and spices to reduce the chance of their being the source of microorganisms in a product, but in many countries use of these is prohibited by legislation. The treatment of fish and meat by exposure to smoke results in several changes that prolong the life of the product: the taking up of various inhibitory substances from the smoke; killing of some spoilage organisms by heat; evaporation of water by the heating, so reducing the a_w.

Although the use of chemicals has been dealt with in this chapter, one must not assume that chemicals act by killing all organisms; some organisms may merely be stopped from growing, so that problems may result if the agents are removed or decay during storage. A good example of this is in the use of nisin in canned foods. It is possible for some endospores to remain dormant for long periods, while the nisin decays, and then to germinate and cause spoilage once the concentration of nisin has fallen to a non-inhibitory level. For this reason all products that incorporate nisin must be treated in some other way sufficiently to control *C. botulinum*.

7.5 Filtration

Bacteria and larger organisms can be removed from otherwise clear liquids by filtration through membranes which have holes with a mean pore size of 0.2 μm. Such treatment will remove spoilage organisms and some pathogens, but will not remove viruses. The use of reverse osmosis (which can be regarded as a form of very fine filtration) in, for example, the desalination of sea water, or ultrafiltration, should remove viruses as well as other microorganisms.

7.6 Combined processes and predictive modelling

There are many advantages to using two or more processes in combination (for example refrigeration of gas-packed foods containing nitrite or heat treatment combined with nisin). Amongst the factors which may be chosen to control the growth and metabolism of microorganisms are: storage temperature; pH; concentration of constituents/additives such as sodium chloride, nitrite, nisin, or organic acid preservatives (e.g. lactic acid, sorbic acid); and gaseous atmosphere. The combination of two or more of these factors often means that the adverse effects on the food are less than if a single process had been used to achieve the same degree of safety or shelf-life. This is because the growth-limiting range of a parameter is generally narrower if other environmental parameters are sub-optimal for the microorganism under consideration. For example, a particular reduction in growth rate can be obtained by use of a lower sodium chloride concentration if the pH is sub-optimal, than would be required at the pH optimal for growth. This well-known principle has often been called the 'hurdle effect'. The principle may be true only for that range of environmental parameters which delineates the boundaries for growth of the organism. Outside these boundaries, where a microorganism is unable to grow, and indeed is likely to die as a result of an inimical environmental factor, sub-optimal values for another environmental parameter may sometimes *increase* survival (i.e. decrease the death rate). Examples of this contrary action have been known for decades. For example, *Salmonella* will die more slowly in the hostile environment of a meat-curing brine when stored at 5°C than when stored at 20°C. The addition of sorbic acid to a system at an a_w of 0.86 has been shown to increase the survival of *Salmonella* at 10°C.

There are so many combinations of the range of possible values for the parameters of preservation processes being operated together that direct testing of all possible combinations for a particular food is usually impracticable. Consequently there has been an increasing interest in developing mathematical modelling computer programs plus databases capable of predicting the response of microorganisms to the process and preservation parameters in a food product. An example of such a project in the UK is the Ministry of Agriculture, Fisheries and Food's food microbiology predictive modelling program for hazardous microorganisms in foods.

The models developed from the input of many growth and survival data must have their predictive value validated. At present food microbiologists have only a limited understanding of the mechanisms by which the environment affects growth and survival, or of the interactive effects on growth and survival of a combination of environmental parameters, or of the interactions that may occur between environmental parameters themselves. An example of the last type of phenomenon is the complex way in which the dissociation constant, pK, of an organic acid preservative such as sorbic acid varies with the a_w (Pethybridge *et al.*, 1983). Another example of an interaction which has been studied is the possible production of a 'Perigo-type' factor when a nitrite-containing system is heated − the inhibitory activity of the system may be an order of magnitude greater than before heating.

It is thus necessary to study not only the interactions of the environmental parameters with the microorganisms, but also the interactions of the environmental parameters with each other. It would be wise to use data-driven models for interpolative predictions only, and not for extrapolation, giving values outside the ranges used to obtain the data on which the models are based. In order to obtain extrapolative power it will be necessary to develop theory-driven models. Whilst models remain essentially data-derived, the food industry must avoid being seduced by what has been described as the 'halo effect' of models – i.e. a model is a 'Good Thing' and therefore its predictions must be right!

8
Legislative aspects

8.1 Introduction

In this chapter we shall look at the principles of the food legislation relating to microbiological quality, with some examples primarily from Great Britain and the USA.

There are often substantial apparent differences in the legislation of various countries, but a closer examination will often reveal that the legislation consists in two parts:

(a) The *primary*, *enabling* legislation. This states the aims and objectives of the particular law. It will usually provide certain wide-ranging general provisions. It will then proceed to provide powers for the relevant Minister or Secretary of State to introduce much more specific Regulations under that Act.

(b) The *Regulations* introduced by the relevant Minister or Secretary of State. These Regulations will state much more specifically the requirements to be met in either the food itself or in its production and handling.

Considered from the point of view of the subject being covered in this book, two different main approaches may be adopted in food-safety or food-quality legislation. Provision for these may be incorporated into either the primary law or regulations, or both.

The legislation may specify particular compositional or microbiological specifications or standards to which food should conform. There would thus be an examination of samples to determine whether batches of food or even individual items of food conform to the requirements.

Alternatively, the legislation may specify the conditions under which food is produced, handled, stored and distributed. This type of legislation may concern itself, for example, with whether food handlers are following appropriate codes of good hygienic or good manufacturing practice. To enforce such legislation, there may be licensing of premises, inspection of premises, approval of a company's codes of Good Manufacturing Practice (GMPs), and monitoring to ensure that GMPs are being properly followed.

These two approaches are very different, and the best consumer protection will be provided by a combination of the two. In addition, a third approach is to provide informative labelling and advice to the consumer on such aspects as storage, proper cooking procedures, etc. Much consumer advice is voluntarily supplied by the food industry; in addition consumer organizations provide a great deal of guidance. However, increasingly, legislation is concerned with ensuring the provision of not only more accurate but also more informative labelling.

8.2 The primary legislation

Food legislation in general has two main objectives:

(a) that the consumer obtains the product which he or she believed was being purchased and that it is of an appropriate quality; and

(b) that the food shall not be harmful to the consumer.

Very early local laws (bylaws) were often enacted to protect the consumer – sometimes on the basis of whether food offered for sale was spoiled, sometimes to limit the period for which food could be offered for sale. For example, the Lord Mayor of London, Dick Whittington (perhaps on the advice of his cat!) instructed his Clerk, J. Carpenter, to collate the then local bylaws of the City of London into the *Liber Albus* (published in 1419). Amongst the bylaws listed were:

> No poulterer, or other person whatsoever, shall expose for sale any manner of poultry that is unsound or unwholesome to man's body, under pain of punishment by the pillory, and the article being burnt under him.

> [A butcher] shall stand to sell his meat there [in the market] in pieces, both small and large, just as he shall please to cut, until high noon; so that by such time he shall have fully made his sale, without getting rid

of any meat, or harbouring it either secretly or openly, or putting it in salt or otherwise. [Any meat that was not sold within the approved period was to be confiscated by the Sheriff].

Early national legislations addressed in particular the subject of adulteration but especially when it caused the food to become harmful, rather than the problems of innate harmful constituents or 'natural contaminants' such as food-poisoning microorganisms. For example, the British *Sale of Food and Drugs Act 1875*, and the USA's *Food and Drugs Act 1906* were primarily aimed at tackling the then widespread problem of food adulteration. Adulterants commonly added by unscrupulous traders up to the end of the nineteenth century were frequently toxic materials. The US *Food and Drugs Act 1906* prohibited the marketing of foods containing added deleterious substances that may render such articles injurious to health. This type of provision remains an important aspect of food law.

As deliberate adulteration of food by the addition of toxic substances lessened, attention turned increasingly to the problems of public-health hazards presented by *natural* food contaminants. Although food-derived chemical poisonings do still sometimes occur, microbial poisoning represents a much more significant concern, and much current legislation is directed at minimizing hazards of a microbial origin.

If a country has a general food law of the type already mentioned, there is theoretically a possibility, where food is microbiologically unsound, of prosecution under a general provision that food shall be of the nature, substance and quality demanded. For example, Section 14 of the British *Food Safety Act 1990* (and the equivalent Section 13 of the *Food Safety [Northern Ireland] Order 1991*) states that 'any person who sells to the purchaser's prejudice any food which is not of the nature or substance or quality demanded by the purchaser shall be guilty of an offence'. However, as pointed out below, prosecutions on this basis are quite likely to fail.

Some primary legislation has included provisions intended to make more explicit the need for food to be 'safe'. For example, Section 8 of the British *Food Safety Act 1990* states that any person is guilty of an offence who sells or offers for sale for human consumption, or has in their possession for such purposes, or transfers to another person for sale, 'any food which fails to comply with safety requirements'. It then states that a food fails to comply with food safety requirements if:

(a) it has been rendered injurious to health by means of [certain operations such as adding a substance to, or abstracting a constituent from, or applying a process];

(b) it is unfit for human consumption; or

(c) it is so contaminated (whether by extraneous matter or otherwise) that it would not be reasonable to expect it to be used for human consumption in that state.

Similarly Section 13 of the Malaysian *Food Act 1983* states that a person commits an offence if they prepare or sell any food that:

(a) has in or upon it any substance which is poisonous, harmful or otherwise injurious to health;

(b) consists in whole or in part of any diseased substance or foreign matter, or is otherwise unfit for human consumption;

(c) is the product of a diseased animal or an animal which has died otherwise than by slaughter;

(d) is the product of a diseased vegetable substance; or

(e) is adulterated.

8.3 Regulations introduced under the primary legislation

A major disadvantage in attempting to bring prosecutions under the general provisions of the primary law is that expert witnesses may be found who have opposing views about, for example, the risk presented to the health of a consumer by a given population of pathogenic microorganisms (or indeed by a given concentration of a harmful chemical). The minimum infective dose of a bacterium such as *Salmonella* will depend on many factors such as the age and general health of the individual consumer and the type of food eaten. If the courts were to interpret such legislation as meaning that the demonstration of either a single pathogenic bacterium or a few molecules of a toxic substance in a kilogram of food offered for sale indicated the commission of an offence, then either consumers would go very hungry, or the food industry would cease to exist, or, much more likely, the law would not be acted upon by the law enforcement officers. The sensitivity of detection of substances such as pesticides or aflatoxin using modern analytical techniques is now so great that some low level of specified injurious substances may be demonstrated in every food sample. Similarly highly sensitive microbiological analytical techniques are now being developed (see Chapter 13).

Consequently, it is more likely that the general provisions of the legislation will be used in prosecutions only in examples of gross abuse, or as part of a long list of offences that include more specific offences of a type which unequivocally can be demonstrated and explained in court. Therefore detailed provisions will be found in Regulations introduced under the powers provided by the primary legislation. An advantage of using such Regulations to cover the more specific aspects, such as food specifications and the related analytical methods or statutory codes of hygienic practice, is that legislatures can permit such Regulations to be introduced rapidly with the minimum of formal proceedings in the legislature. Thus the empowered Minister can quickly take action on any recommendations from his scientific advisers that relate to such things as rapidly emerging new public health problems, improvements in our understanding of problems, or improvements in analytical techniques. Regulations may concern such things as:

(1) compositional or microbiological standards or specifications for the foods themselves;

(2) hygienic precautions to be taken during preparation, storage and/or distribution;

(3) processing procedures or processing parameters such as the heat treatment to be applied during thermal processing;

(4) the training or qualifications required of food handlers, food manufacturers and the like;

(5) the design, construction and licensing of food premises;

(6) the training and qualifications required of enforcement officers, food analysts, etc.;

(7) procedures for inspections, seizure and recall of food, closure of premises, prosecutions, etc.

8.4 Microbiological standards or specifications for foods

Microbiological standards or specifications for foods may be introduced into a country's law. A correctly drawn up specification would include:

1. A statement of the microorganisms or microbial toxins of concern.

2. A description of the sampling plan to be applied to obtain the samples to be examined (see Chapter 14).

3. The microbiological limits (concentration of microorganism or toxin per unit quantity of food) appropriate to the food and its intended market.

4. The precise analytical method to be employed, including, for example, the methods of sub-sampling and preparation of dilutions, the medium to be employed, the source of medium or constituents, the incubation temperature and time. Examples of standardized analytical procedures are given in Chapter 12.

There may already exist in a country a recognized source of standard methodology – for example the British Standards referred to in Chapter 12, or the Bacteriological Analytical Manual of the US Federal Food and Drugs Administration, published by the Association of Official Analytical Chemists (AOAC). In this case it may be sufficient to name in the legislation the appropriate standard analytical method to be used. For example, the British *Milk (Special Designation) Regulations 1989* specifies that the coliform test be carried out according to *British Standard 4285: Section 3.7:1987*, and the aerobic mesophilic count according to *British Standard 4285: Section 2.1: 1984*. Alternatively, a country lacking its own nationally recognized standard methodology for a particular test could refer in its legislation to some internationally recognized method (for example an ISO method such as those mentioned in Chapter 12). In the absence of any such work of reference that is acceptable to the legislators for the particular analytical method required, it will be necessary to describe the detail of the method in the legislation. For example, the British *Milk-based Drinks (Hygiene and Heat Treatment) Regulations 1983* specified that the coliform test to be carried out on pasteurized milk-based drink must be performed using quarter-strength Ringer's solution and brilliant green lactose bile salts broth, with the recipes for the medium, and all other aspects being described in the Regulations.

Legislation may describe the microbiological quality in fairly simple terms in the context of the maximum count permissible in a sample, with the description of the conditions under which the samples are to be taken, and the number to be taken, being separated from the quality specification itself or even omitted from the legislation. For example, in the British *Milk (Special Designation) Regulations 1989* untreated milk is required to have a coliform count of less than 100 ml^{-1} and an aerobic mesophilic count of not more than 20 000 ml^{-1}. In some countries legislation incorporating microbiological specifications has sometimes introduced a 'zero-tolerance level' for pathogens. However, these are in many ways unreasonable provisions to place into law. For example, *Salmonella* is widespread in wild animals as well as in farm and domestic animals, so that it is unreasonable to expect a trader to be able to supply raw poultry or meat guaranteed free from *Salmonella*, particularly when there are no non-destructive methods of microbiological examination of food which could enable 100 % inspection to take place. Consequently, current legislative provisions in those countries possessing statutory microbiological end-product specifications are usually now drawn up in a manner that recognizes the probabilistic nature of sampling and analysis. Such specifications will often be presented within a framework of 2-class and 3-class sampling plans similar to those recommended by ICMSF (see Chapter 14). The threshold populations of target microorganisms described in such specifications must take into account such aspects as the minimum infective or toxic dose for the target consumers and the subsequent storage and treatment of such food. Thus low concentrations of salmonellae might be permissible in raw poultry or meat since these raw foods should be cooked before consumption. High concentrations would however be unacceptable since they suggest either that the meat has come from animals suffering from massive systemic infection or that the storage of the raw meat has permitted multiplication of the salmonellae; furthermore they would carry a much greater hazard in respect of possible cross-contamination of cooked foods from the raw foods. Thus microbiological specifications for foods should not be introduced into legislation without very careful consideration of all the sociological, financial, epidemiological and even political implications of the numerical values proposed for the microbiological counts.

In a number of countries the incidence of human listeriosis has appeared to be increasing in recent years (see Chapter 4). Recent surveys in many countries have demonstrated that *Listeria monocytogenes* is common in foods. Since the organism is an ubiquitous psychrotroph it is not feasible to demand that all foods on sale shall be *free* from *L. monocytogenes*. However, once a number of unknowns, such as minimum infective dose, have been determined it should be possible eventually to specify the maximum permissible concentration of viable listeriae in certain foods. Because of the destructive nature of microbiological testing this would not remove all risk of contracting human listeriosis from foods but it could reduce it to an acceptably low level of probability. Increasingly legislators are looking towards this *de minimis* approach to risks, whether from food additives such as food preservatives, or contaminants such as pesticide residues. For example 'safe' would be defined to mean that 'there is a reasonable certainty that the risks are negligible under the intended conditions of use'. It would seem reasonable to take a similar line on microbiological quality parameters.

8.5 Hygienic production and handling of foods

Official inspection of premises and samples cannot *guarantee* that all production is of a given quality, and government enforcement officers should act as the external auditors of systems of management for safety and quality established and monitored by the qualified technical staff within each food business. Such an approach not only encourages the higher levels of efficiency and safety which can be reached by a well-motivated self-regulatory quality management system, but also enables enforcement officers to use their resources most effectively.

Very extensive Regulations of this type are in some cases introduced under the primary enabling legislation. For example, in the USA in the late 1960s the first Codes of Good Manufacturing Practice (GMPs) were issued under Section 701(a) of the *Federal Food, Drug and Cosmetic Act 1938*. There are now many such GMPs published as part of the *Code of Federal Regulations*; additions to, and changes in, these CFRs appear in the Federal Register. Examples of such GMPs are CFR Part 110: 'Current good manufacturing practices in manufacturing, packing or holding human foods', and CFR Part 113: 'Thermally processed low-acid foods packaged in hermetically sealed containers'.

8.6 Labelling of foods and advice to consumers

Brown (1989) suggested that warning statements are particularly useful when the product presents a hazard to a specific minority of the population – for example in the context of allergic response to a food additive, or in the greater susceptibility of pregnant women to *Listeria monocytogenes*. He also pointed out that warnings or cautions on labels could provide a way for a regulatory agency to deal with a problem that involves difficult political decisions.

8.6.1 Labels incorporating warning notices

Much food poisoning is caused by cross-contamination within the domestic kitchen of cooked foods by microorganisms deriving from food materials such as raw meat and raw poultry. It has been suggested that raw meat and poultry should be labelled in such a way as to emphasize the possibility that it may contain pathogens, together with advice to the consumer on ways to minimize the risks from cross-contamination.

The British *Milk (Special Designation) Regulations 1989* require untreated (i.e. raw) milk offered for sale to be labelled 'This milk has not been heat-treated and may therefore contain organisms harmful to health'.

8.6.2 'Use by' dates

The inclusion in the label on perishable foods of a 'use by' date helps to inform the consumer of the likely safe storage period for the food. For example, the European Community's *Food Labelling Directive 89/395/EEC amending Food Labelling Directive 79/1 12/EEC* requires highly perishable prepacked foods which could, after a fairly short storage period, constitute a danger to health to be labelled with 'use by' dates together with a description of the storage conditions to be used. Obviously, any microbiological specification established in relation to food sampled at the time and place of production needs to take into account the proposed storage life; indeed, in some legislated microbiological specifications it is possible to see two sets of microbiological counts being specified – the first to apply to food as at the time of sampling at the place of production, the second to apply to the food after a specified storage period at a stated storage temperature.

8.6.3 Cooking instructions

If a particular hazard exists from food poisoning because of the likelihood of inadequate cooking, advice may be offered to the consumer on these aspects. For example, the label on prepacked frozen poultry could indicate clearly and unambiguously the defrosting and cooking procedures to be applied. Once again, this advice may be provided by government information services or voluntarily by the industry. It could, however, also be required by legislation.

9

Modern approaches to quality management

9.1 Definition of quality and of quality management

Quality is not absolute. It has to be quantified and clearly defined for individual purposes, in which considerations of cost and reliability will be included. Quality is often defined in terms of 'fitness for use'. The definition provided in the relevant International Standard (*ISO 8402:1986*, or the equivalent *BS 4778:1987*) states that quality is 'the totality of features and characteristics of a product or service that bear on its ability to satisfy stated or implied needs'. Food of good microbiological quality thus should be organoleptically acceptable and remain so to the end of the stated shelf life, and should be safe in respect of food poisoning organisms and organisms capable of causing foodborne disease. The range of laboratory investigations used for the purpose of monitoring these quality parameters will be discussed in Chapters 12 and 13. Costing of the product must take adequate account of the cost of appropriate monitoring.

Since all microbiological methods of analysis so far developed are destructive of the product examined, it is not possible to provide consumer protection against the receipt of defective product by carrying out microbiological examinations of all end-products to judge end-product quality against an end-product specification. (The nature of end-product specifications will be discussed in Chapter 14.) It is important therefore that the food industry (and indeed governments) approach the problem by attempting to ensure that there is a quality management system operating within the food manufacturing, distribution and retailing chain.

Traditionally quality has been regarded as the responsibility of the 'Quality Control (QC) Department'. However, for the industry to meet the consumer demand for better quality products, it is necessary to adopt a comprehensive approach that organizes and involves the entire workforce from the managing director down. The importance of this is underlined by *ISO 8402:1986* defining quality policy as 'the overall quality intentions and direction of an organization as regards quality, as formally expressed by top management'. This is just as important in today's markets as is the company having a well-defined marketing strategy. Indeed a number of the more successful food-manufacturing and food-retailing companies have incorporated quality policy statements into their marketing approach, so that the consumer has come to link their name with the concept of high quality. For example, in the UK, many consumers are prepared to pay more for food from Marks and Spencer food stores because they perceive M & S to be synonymous with 'high quality', even though the ordinary consumer is not informed of the detailed microbiological specifications and codes of hygienic practice in food manufacture that M & S require their suppliers to meet.

To achieve good microbiological quality, it is essential for all workers to receive appropriate training in hygiene. One of the problems in many food manufacturing and food processing factories is that much of the work is seasonal, so that unskilled temporary and casual labour may represent the majority of the workforce at certain times of the year. Companies truly committed to a system of total quality management will nevertheless ensure that even casual and temporary workers are not involved in food handling until they have received adequate training in hygiene and are positively motivated to hygienic production methods.

9.2 Total quality management systems

In the electronic, electrical and mechanical engineering industries, several philosophical approaches have been proposed by various quality consultants, with their own systems of obtaining improvements in quality. Three consultants often quoted are Crosby, Deming and Juran. However, some of these approaches which may work well in such industries seem to be less applicable to the microbiological quality of food. For example, in Crosby's philosophy there is no place for statistically acceptable levels of quality. In his view, as soon as a manufacturer accepts the possibility of some of the output being defective in respect of a particular quality criterion, then there is a danger that the workforce will tend to regard *this lower* quality as the norm, and adjust working practices accordingly. He therefore argues that there is only one performance standard that should be applied – namely *zero defects*. This approach may seem reasonable for a factory producing, for example, television sets, every one of which can be non-destructively tested. It is more difficult to put into practice in a food factory producing 100 000 items per day, particularly because microbiological examination of an item involves its destruction and therefore denies it to the consumer. Although Crosby's zero defect approach cannot be used in end-product specifications for foods, nevertheless, the philosophy of *wishing* to achieve zero defects can be adopted by seeking to identify and control all hazards that exist in the food and in the food production process. This concept is the subject of Chapter 16.

Other approaches seem to be more directly applicable to the food industry. For example, Deming defined quality as 'a predictable degree of uniformity and dependability, at low cost and suited to the market'. In his view, 'statistical control does not imply the absence of defective items, but is a state of random variation in which the limits of variation are predictable'. Deming's approach seems to fit in well with the idea of having end-product specifications which include appropriate acceptance sampling plans (to be discussed in Chapter 14), but it is as well not to overlook the fact that a food could conform to an end-product specification and yet provide a substantial public-health risk, perhaps because the possible presence of a particular pathogen has not been recognized for that food. In this context Juran's view of quality as 'fitness for use or purpose' is an important one; Juran distinguished this from 'conformance to specification'. Juran pointed out over 30 years ago that a product could meet all the specifications applied to it, and yet be dangerous in use. It is not sufficiently recognized that the fulfilling of a specification carries no valid implications for factors not specifically examined. For example, the uninitiated may judge a batch of raw milk to be of high microbiological quality because it displays low counts on both plate count agar and violet red bile agar; yet such milk could be laden with *Mycobacterium bovis*, *Coxiella burnetii*,

Brucella abortus, *Leptospira*, tickborne encephalitis virus or other pathogens. In recent years there have been a number of examples in food microbiology that have demonstrated this point only too well. This justifies the ISO definition of quality as relating to fitness of use rather than to conformance to specification.

Crosby, Deming, Juran and all other quality consultants, while they may differ in their approach to quality, agree that a successful quality management system will be achieved only when there is a total commitment by *top management*, and that in a factory failing to achieve good quality the fault lies primarily with senior management and not with the workers on the factory floor.

9.3 Quality assurance and quality control

The internationally agreed definitions provided in *ISO 8402:1986* are:

Quality assurance – 'all those planned and systematic actions necessary to provide adequate confidence that a product or service will satisfy given requirements for quality'.

Quality control – 'the operational techniques and activities that are used to fulfil requirements for quality'.

Quality control is therefore one component of an integrated system of quality assurance.

9.4 Codes of Good Manufacturing Practice

Within the food factory there should be management procedures aimed at the application of Codes of Good Manufacturing Practice (CGMP). Suitable Outline Guides for CGMP may be published as advisory booklets by government departments (e.g. HMSO, 1989), or by the relevant professional institutions (e.g. IFST, 1987, 1990). Individual food companies will then need to incorporate these guidelines into company-specific and factory-specific CGMP.

Food hygiene legislation may be aimed at policing the conformance to recognized CGMP. In the UK, it has been usual for any advisory CGMP published by the Government to be separate from the legislation and *not* to have force in a court of law, whereas in the USA, federal CGMP have been regarded as legally enforceable.

9.5 End-product specifications

With the increase in international trade in food products rather than merely primary agricultural products, it has become necessary for importing and exporting countries to agree on appropriate end-product specifications operated within reliable acceptance sampling plans. Since the objective of an acceptance sampling plan is to provide the basis for a decision on whether to accept or to reject a batch of food, it is obvious that there is an implied element of quality control in the sense that intervention can prevent 'unacceptable' batches from passing through to the consumer. However, there is no application of quality control on the food production process itself, although conformance or nonconformance of a food product to its specification can provide monitoring information about the entire history of the food material up to the point of sampling (and in this sense is fulfilling a 'quality assurance' function).

Nevertheless, as already pointed out, microbiological analyses destroy the product, and consequently end-product examination cannot provide the consumer with total quality assurance in respect of the item actually purchased and consumed. An equally valid approach to providing the consumer with adequate protection against receiving a poor-quality product is to monitor and control the production, processing and distribution system, usually by the application of a Code of Good Manufacturing Practice. For some time it has been recognized that an internationally agreed standard for a quality management system would be of great value in indicating that appropriate CGMP were being applied. In recent years many food manufacturing companies, especially those interested in developing their international trade, have been seeking official certification of their factories under *ISO 9000/1/2/3/4:1987* (equivalent to the UK's standard *BS 5750:1987*). This will be discussed further in Chapter 10.

9.6 Use of laboratory investigations and the statistical analysis of results

There are different approaches that can be adopted in the statistical analysis of results. The different techniques will prove most useful in different sets of circumstances.

We can identify three types of laboratory:

1. *Laboratories concerned with the examination of samples of end-product* for the purpose of determining the quality of a given batch or lot, probably to compare these results against a published statutory or guideline end-product specification. Such laboratories will include those of governmental control agencies, port authorities, and also industrial laboratories if, for example, the manufacturer wishes to check batch quality against either an 'in-house' specification or a government specification. In such laboratories a decision may cause a substantial financial penalty to result (e.g. if a batch or shipment is condemned). Consequently the number of samples drawn from the batch is chosen in such a way as to provide a specified confidence in the reliability of the result. These investigations into the conformance to specification are undertaken within an *acceptance sampling plan* and are the basis of the publication by the International Commission on Microbiological Specifications for Foods (ICMSF) *Micro-organisms in Foods Vol. II* (Chapter 14).

2. *Laboratories concerned with the examination of relatively few types of product*, for example, laboratories in milk processing and bottling plants or canning factories. In such laboratories a large number of samples from each product type can be examined over a period. *Trends* in counts which occur over time, although the samples have been drawn from different batches, may reflect trends of a deterioration or improvement in hygiene, for example. To detect such trends *control charts* can be used (Chapter 15).

3. *Laboratories concerned with the examination of a wide variety of food types from many production systems, which are not producing the same food type continuously over an extended period*. An example of such a laboratory would be that of a large hotel chain which monitors the output of the various hotel kitchens. In such cases it will not be possible to apply control charts, and the only statistical analysis of results possible will be the use of *confidence interval* calculations on individual plate counts, MPN counts, etc. in order to determine not only the confidence one can have in the individual result, but also to give an indication of the extent to which laboratory procedures are in statistical control (Chapter 15). The general aspects of quality assurance checks on laboratory activities will be discussed in Chapters 10 and 16.

In addition, any laboratories involved in the monitoring of hygienic procedures and inspections of factories to determine their conformance with CGMP may frequently take samples from various points in the production line. These samples may be of food constituents, partially processed food, swabs and rinses of processing equipment, etc., which will be studied to determine if they are of a suitable standard. The results obtained can then be used to interpret observations made in the factory in terms of their microbiological implications. When using the data in this way, it can often be of value to determine the confidence intervals on the counts.

Some practical aspects of quality management

10.1 The International Organization for Standardization guidelines on quality management systems and quality assurance standards – *ISO 9000* series

Recently there has been a major change in attitude towards the attainment of a uniform quality for a product. It has been recognized that uniform quality cannot be assured merely by end-product testing by a 'quality control' department. It is necessary for the whole workforce to be involved in the desire and the effort to attain the particular quality that has been decided upon by product designers and marketing personnel. Means of changing and maintaining appropriate attitudes and procedures amongst workforces in the manufacturing and service industries by quality systems have been addressed by a number of standards. The *ISO 9000/9001/9002/9003:1987* series of publications (to which the European Standards EN29000 series and the British Standard – *BS 5750:1987* are equivalent) is a series of standards describing the requirements for a quality system within industry. It is not industry-specific and it does not aim to impose any specific quality system. The *ISO 9000* series also deals with the need to establish procedures which can lead to between-laboratory and between-country confidence in quality standards which have been agreed between parties.

To be successful in the modern world a company must recognize that customers are increasingly sophisticated in their requirements with respect to the quality of products. It must put in place mechanisms to define these expectations and to involve the whole workforce in striving to achieve these expectations. It must arrange to monitor materials, production, packaging, storage and distribution procedures, as well as the products themselves. To facilitate trade between companies and between countries it is necessary to establish procedures for ensuring the professional standard of the quality management associated with each product line. Therefore companies have to establish a suitable *quality system* ('The organizational structure, responsibilities, procedures, processes and resources for implementing quality management') and to make available adequate equipment, personnel and other resources to effect the quality system. Certification schemes independent of the companies must be available to approve factory manuals and to see that stated procedures are known and practised by all relevant members of the workforce. Becoming certificated under one of the *ISO 9000* standards signifies that the company has adopted a quality policy, set in place a quality system, that it has developed and recorded all the procedures necessary to achieve this for all the products being manufactured under the certification scheme, and that it has in place an internal audit system to ensure that the requisite procedures are followed. In other words, in order to gain certification for a product line the company has to present written evidence that it knows how to manufacture the product under a system of quality management *and* it has to show that it is doing it.

Each standard addresses a different range of activities of the supplier: e.g. design, production, storage and delivery of the product (ISO 9001); or production, storage and delivery (ISO 9002). It is necessary to determine which of these standards is appropriate to the situation.

10.2 What type of assurance about quality do the supplier and customer need?

Assuring that a product is of a certain quality requires that what is meant by *quality* should be defined for that particular product (Chapter 9) through implicit or explicit agreement between the supplier and the customer. In deciding on the nature of assessments to be made, factors to be considered will include: the extent to which any production procedure and product already have an established record of reliability; the number of stages that the product has to go through during its 'manufacture'; the extent of the safety risk associated with a faulty product; and the need to provide a product that is not so expensive as to be uneconomic. For many products a large responsibility for detecting real and perceived requirements of potential customers will fall on the marketing staff, who will need to assess the market potential with respect to grade of quality required, size of market, etc. so that the economics of making a product at a specified grade can be evaluated. These staff will also be involved in the test marketing of such new products and must review quality aspects such as adequacy of distribution and storage facilities, relevant training of retail staff, etc. Results of various assessments, which will include the producer's verification and possibly some outside organization's verification, of the supplier's assessment procedures, will need to be documented.

10.3 The essential components of a quality system

Reference to the *ISO 9000* series should be made for general guidance on the various components of quality systems as they apply in any industry for any product. Here we consider some of the points in the context of the food industry.

10.3.1 Responsibility for quality

Responsibility for attaining a required quality of a product lies with *all* members of the company. The positive attitude to quality must pervade the whole workforce from the managing director to the packer and delivery worker. Workers dealing with specific processes can become involved in discussions on changes to improve quality and even in writing the relevant parts of factory manuals produced for certification, so that a move to embrace the quality system procedures requires collaboration between members of the workforce at all levels and in fact stimulates such collaboration. The workforce comes to realize the advantages of having a disciplined approach to quality management with good communication between workers, good documentation and control of documents, and clearly defined duties and responsibilities.

All workers must be receptive to the value of customer feedback in the form of complaints or other aspects of customer experience and expectations. Workers involved in the design of new products must consider quality requirements from the first stages of planning, including such aspects as resilience to storage and likely methods for monitoring quality.

The increasing availability of predictive models to anticipate the biostatic or biocidal effects of various combinations of methods for controlling microorganisms is facilitating the choice of optimum formulation, processing and storage procedures to assure from a very early stage of design development that the product will be of good quality. Hazard analysis and critical control point procedures (HACCP, Chapter 16) are developed to choose the *relevant* monitoring procedures relative to the *appropriate* organism(s) and the correct functioning of plant, at the *correct* stages of the manufacturing and distribution processes.

Maintenance staff, clerks and others, who may not see themselves as being directly involved in the product, must be just as much concerned with the quality of their work as must the workforce more obviously directly involved in producing goods. Their inefficiency might have a direct effect on the quality of the product, through failure to repair some production-line machinery correctly or to order a correct material, etc. For example, failure to maintain a chlorination plant for water used to cool canned foods can lead to a major outbreak of typhoid, and use of plastic film of incorrect gas permeability characteristics can reduce the quality of gas-packed foods. Furthermore low quality of work by any member of a company means that, through such inefficient work, products are unnecessarily expensive to the customer and are therefore of reduced quality since cost is an important factor in determining the perception of the quality of products.

To achieve involvement of the whole workforce in quality it is necessary to develop and to state clearly the policies, and to establish the responsibilities and rewards of individual workers. Such policies and responsibilities must not be in conflict with company policies dealing with other matters or with other duties of individuals. For example, the cost of quality assurance must be realistically included in costing of the product and must be seen as an *investment*. Larger sales are likely to result from the raising of customer appreciation of the reliability of the product. Losses will be reduced because there will be less waste and fewer production-line stoppages, and greater resilience of the product to criteria and problems imposed external to the company. Incentive bonus payment schemes for workers must not encourage 'short-cuts' of a sort that jeopardize the quality of the product. Furthermore, the requirement for workers when suffering from an infection not to work at certain points on a production line must not be in conflict with payment policy – those workers reporting infections must not be financially disadvantaged as a result of being suspended from work or being transferred to other work.

10.3.2 The need for training and provision of facilities

Involvement of all the workforce in assuring quality of products requires adequate training, including maintenance of standards by refresher courses and courses associated with introduction of new products and procedures. Some sectors of the food industry have traditionally relied on unskilled and seasonal workers, making training a considerable challenge, but such difficulties cannot be used as an excuse for poor understanding amongst workers. Either the training must be extensive and followed by appropriate financial rewards to those attaining the required standard, or management must specify and limit the demand of duties and working procedures in such a simple manner that in all cases the standard of dedication and knowledge required is appropriate for the worker and the task that he or she has to undertake. Such action may involve the provision of more sophisticated machinery that demands less of the workers or that requires fewer, but more highly paid, workers. Specific instructions regarding working procedures and definitions of relevant aspects of good workmanship should be available to production-line workers and presented in an appropriate form, making use of simple unambiguous language and relevant pictures.

10.3.3 The need to define responsibilities

Top management is responsible for ensuring that each member of the workforce has his or her duties and responsibilities clearly defined and that he or she knows the company policy on quality. Those who work on, or supervise, a particular process must not be those responsible to management for reporting on quality assessment of the product of the process, because conflicts of interests may arise such as the temptation to maintain production through judicious choice of quality-assurance procedures, sampling plans, etc. that minimize the chance of detecting faulty products. Nevertheless, pervading all aspects of quality management should be the realization that identification of actual or potential problems relating to poor quality, and efficient action to alleviate such problems, improve the quality of the product, its consumer acceptability and therefore the competitiveness of the company. All aspects of quality must be adequately monitored and controlled.

10.3.4 Reliable procedures for quality assessment

First it must be decided what types of features are to be monitored in order for the quality of a product to be assessed and at what stages of production and distribution such monitoring shall occur (Chapter 16). Then the specific method for monitoring each feature must be chosen. For example, it may be decided to monitor shelf life of a product. How will this be done? Let us assume that it is decided that part of the assessment of the quality of a product will be to store samples from the production line for a given time at a given temperature and then to count the numbers of some particular component of the microbial flora of the product so that on the basis of the results obtained a decision will be taken about whether an appropriate quality has been achieved. In order for such a monitoring procedure to be reliable a number of criteria must be fulfilled, including the relevance of the monitoring procedure chosen. Of particular importance here is the reliability of the procedures, and the recording and general aspects of interpretation of the results obtained. It is necessary to ensure: that the procedure for choosing samples for examination is clearly laid down and followed; that the storage conditions are specified; that the temperature control for the storage is checked in some appropriate manner at appropriately frequent time intervals to see that it is functioning correctly; and that the procedure for assessing microbial load after storage is standardized. Factors requiring attention in order to ensure standardization of a method for assessment of microbial load include: developing a uniform manipulative technique amongst staff, requiring adequate training and careful supervision; using controls to ensure that growth media are of an appropriate type for the organisms being counted, and of a standard composition, samples being regularly checked for performance; and regular checking of incubator temperatures using an instrument that itself is regularly checked. Unless reliability is built into the monitoring procedure by the establishment and maintenance of such procedures, the maintenance of quality is not assured because the means of monitoring that quality are not assured.

10.3.5 The recording of data relating to quality assurance

Procedures must be decided and rigidly followed for the making and storage of appropriate records. Such records will be useful to the company for a variety of purposes but may also be important for consultation by, for example, agencies of the governments of the producing country and receiving country, etc. They will also be required in the event of legal proceedings in order to show that all reasonable steps were taken to ensure that the product was of a good quality (a 'due diligence' defence). Records to be kept must include temperature charts of HTST and UHT treatments, canning retorts, cold rooms, etc., reports on routine testing of equipment, and audit reports (Section 10.3.6). They must relate to specific batches of product, which must be marked with a batch identification code.

10.3.6 *The need to establish and maintain the credibility of the quality system*

Procedures must be established in the company for auditing the quality system that management has put in place. Such audits must be carried out regularly by persons not involved in the procedures being monitored. Audit staff much check that the rôles and duties of all concerned with the product and its monitoring are clearly understood by all and that training and record keeping are as required. The results of such audits must be considered by senior management, who must ensure that any recommendations for improvement following the audits are put into effect.

If the procedures for maintaining and monitoring the quality of a product are to have credibility outside the company, the procedures of the factory and of the quality-assurance laboratory must be approved by independent assessors. Such assessment helps to achieve uniformity between laboratories in standards of professionalism and reliability of results (*not necessarily uniformity of choice of procedure*). To fulfil the requirements of *ISO 9000*, a system of certification by independent inspectors should be established by government or some other appropriate agency (a UK system is called the National Measurement Accreditation Scheme, NAMAS). Negotiations between governments are required to ensure that accreditation schemes in different countries achieve an international conformity. The relevant European standard for the accreditation of laboratories is *EN 45000*.

The establishment of clearly defined procedures must not be allowed to stifle legitimate and agreed changes in procedures that have been shown to improve the standard of quality or procedures for monitoring quality. When the customer of the company is a supermarket chain or some other informed body, possibly with its own laboratory for assessing quality, it will be necessary to come to a clearly defined agreement on the criteria of quality to be applied and on the methods for verification of the quality. This will require, for example, agreement on the type of microorganism to be monitored, the statistical statement of the standard required (see Chapter 14), and the choice of reagents and procedures to be used for detecting the agreed type of microorganism (see Chapters 12 and 13).

10.3.7 Quality management in production and distribution

The *ISO 9000* series specifies a variety of aspects of quality management and quality assurance relating to production, storage and delivery. Such aspects are considered in the context of food in other chapters of the book and are covered adequately by a consideration of the Hazard Analysis and Critical Control Point (HACCP) approach to the provision of microbiologically safe and wholesome food (Chapter 16).

11

The design and management of a food microbiology laboratory

11.1 The need for concern

A badly designed and badly run microbiology laboratory is a dangerous place both for those who work in it and for others. Many microbiological procedures involve great amplification of the pathogens in a sample in order to detect them in routine analyses: for example, in order to detect one or a few salmonellae in a sample of chicken the number of these organisms is deliberately increased to many millions. Thus, the laboratory can become a major source of pathogens, making it important to minimize the opportunity for contamination to be released in the laboratory or to be spread from the laboratory to the factory. There is also the very real risk that the laboratory can be the cause of contamination of samples brought in for examination – careless handling of cultures from a positive sample can contaminate other samples in the laboratory so that truly negative samples will be recorded as positive, leading to much anxiety and unnecessary expense. There are, of course, chemical and physical hazards in microbiological laboratories as in other laboratories, and these also require attention. It therefore behoves those who provide laboratories for microbiologists, and those who work in the laboratories, to ensure that the work proceeds safely and the risk of contamination is minimized. All too often inexperienced workers set to work in inadequate laboratories without being provided with adequate supervision and support.

Senior management should ensure that government guidelines and regulations relating to the design and functioning of laboratories under their control are met, and that detailed written local safety rules are issued to laboratory staff and others, such as security staff, as appropriate. Specialists in the design of laboratories and the provision of laboratory facilities should be involved. People who are to work in the laboratories should be involved in the planning stage and should monitor the design because it is unlikely that the designers will have a complete grasp of what is required in each particular establishment. This chapter introduces some of the points that should be considered, the prime purposes being to alert managers and laboratory workers to the importance that must be attached to the provision of laboratory facilities, and to help in improving standards of laboratory facilities and safety. All members of the organization have to be imbued with the desire to make the laboratory a safe place for all workers and to ensure that it does not pose a threat to the environment or the general public. Disciplinary procedures for failure to follow safe practices should be in place and widely publicized.

There is a marked difference in attitudes to safety at work in different countries. In some, legislation is not sufficiently specific, so that responsibility is diffuse and no individual can readily be held responsible for failures in safety procedures. In others, failure to ensure a safe working environment may result in fining and imprisonment of individuals, thus creating an atmosphere in which everyone comes to see that attention to safety matters is part of a professional approach to their work.

Throughout this chapter the term 'laboratory' is used to denote one or a collection of rooms associated with the practical scientific study, particularly microbiological study, of foods and their ingredients. We have used the term 'should', rather than 'must', in connection with safety instructions, because it is for local organizations and relevant government agencies in the country of work to decide whether the imperative is to be used in connection with any particular item. Nevertheless in no case have we made recommendations that should be set aside without careful consideration of the relevant legislation, the local situation, and the risks involved.

11.2 Siting and servicing of the laboratory

Because the microbiological laboratory is potentially a source of contamination of food products, it should be sited in such a way that unauthorized movement of laboratory staff to the production and distribution areas, and of production workers to the laboratory, is impracticable. The entry to the laboratory should be separate from the entry to the production and distribution area, and laboratory staff should wear distinctive clothing. Ideally, samples for analysis from the factory should be taken and delivered by persons who do not enter the laboratory. If the use of laboratory staff for sampling is unavoidable, utmost care should be taken to minimize the risk of transfer of organisms from the laboratory to the production area – washing of hands should be thorough, and separate overalls and footwear, stored away from the laboratory, should be worn when the production area is visited.

Hand-washing facilities should be provided within the laboratory. Sinks should be designated specifically for the purpose so that no one is deterred from washing hands because other work is being done or a sink contains apparatus. Taps and soap dispensers should be provided with wrist, elbow or foot operation to minimize the risk of transfer of contamination from dirty hands to clean hands.

Ventilation of the laboratory should be arranged so that air from the laboratory cannot pass to other areas of the building. This aspect is particularly important if mechanical ventilation is used. In order to minimize the chance of microbes being passed from the laboratory, the design and balance of the air-handling system should be such that more air is extracted to the outside than is deliberately fed in. Thus, the laboratory should be under negative pressure compared with other areas of the building. This regime should not be disturbed by the switching on of booster extract fans in non-laboratory areas. Thought should be given to possible 'out of hours' working by laboratory staff, when factory air supply may be switched off, so possibly nullifying arrangements made for the laboratory to be at negative pressure relative to the factory. Air from the laboratory should not be passed by ventilation systems to other areas of the building but should be vented to the outside. Filtration of the exhausted air to remove any released organisms should not be necessary, except in the case of safety cabinets, which should be used for any work carrying a considerable risk of the release of a large amount of aerosol of a potentially pathogenic organism (Section 11.5).

Fume cupboards and safety cabinets should be sited in positions away from main passageways in the room. They should be put where air inlets to, or outlets from, the laboratory will not disturb the patterns of air currents established by these items for the minimization of contamination. The air supply to the laboratory should be such that there is no risk of a safety cabinet drawing contaminated air from a fume cupboard or vice versa, as a result of their air extract demands. Similarly, there should be no risk of air being drawn from other laboratories via a corridor or other communal area when one of the items is switched on.

Water should not be fed from the mains directly to the laboratory because of the risk of contamination spreading back from the laboratory to other areas served by the water, but should come from a tank.

Cut-off points for water and gas should be prominently sited and marked so as to be readily accessible in the event of an emergency. Electricity should be supplied through some form of circuit breaker that operates automatically in the event of a dangerous situation arising but it may be practicable to have incubators, refrigerators, computer monitors, etc. on a separate circuit from bench equipment so that no more equipment than necessary is interrupted in the event of a hazard developing.

Transfer of data to production areas should be by telephone, computer links or other electronic means to ensure that no written reports can carry contamination from the laboratory.

11.3 Assessing the risk of the proposed work and establishing appropriate facilities and working procedures

The principle already stated, that material should not go from the laboratory to food production areas, means that production of starter cultures or other materials to be used in a food production process should not be undertaken in a microbiology laboratory involved in product testing. Risks associated with the type of work to be undertaken should be assessed in an informed and formal manner. In fact some governments *require* that this is done and that written records are kept of such assessments. All substances to be used – chemicals, microorganisms and other biological materials – should be considered in the context of the use to which they are to be put, of the hazards they carry, and of the procedures required to minimize these hazards. Because the laboratories we are considering are associated with food production, guidelines for the categorization of pathogens in clinical laboratories may be insufficiently rigorous.

11.4 Assessing microbiological risk and deciding on appropriate control measures

Four categories of microorganisms with respect to risk to health are generally recognized:

(1) those that pose no known hazard;

(2) those that may be widespread in the community and that have some known hazard but are unlikely in the laboratory situation to affect healthy adults who have been specifically trained and who are directed by a competent microbiologist;

(3) those that are not common in the community and that may cause serious disease as a result of inhalation or skin penetration;

(4) those that are life-threatening to anyone coming into contact with them.

Each category of microorganism should be worked on in a laboratory of appropriate standard with appropriate equipment, detailed guidance being obtainable from sources listed in the bibliography or from relevant government agencies. The food microbiology laboratory should be designed, equipped and run on the assumption that it will deal with category 2 organisms (e.g. *Escherichia coli*, *Campylobacter*, *Staphylococcus*, *Listeria*, most *Salmonella*) unless there are specific considerations of dangers in the context of the food industry (e.g. *Clostridium botulinum*, which, because of the extremely serious risk in the event of contamination of processed foods, should not be deliberately cultivated in a food microbiology laboratory) and that no work will be deliberately undertaken with category 3 organisms (e.g. *Mycobacterium tuberculosis*, *M. bovis*, *Shigella dysenteriae* type 1, *Salmonella typhi*, *Brucella*). Problems relating to toxins should be considered in the context of chemicals (Section 11.6). Category 2 organisms can generally be studied on the open bench but any process likely to generate an extensive aerosol (e.g. vigorous blending) should be undertaken in a safety cabinet or in some other apparatus specifically designed to contain the aerosol. Use of large quantities of category 2 organisms or performance of experiments obviously carrying an increased risk of infection should be carried out under conditions appropriate for category 3 organisms.

Some workers do not like to keep stock cultures of any pathogens in a food microbiology laboratory but in our view this is not logical.

Media and procedures should be tested periodically with known positive samples containing stock cultures to confirm their efficiency. Furthermore, several procedures used to isolate organisms from foods can result in very large numbers of pathogens, far more than might be present in a stock culture.

Legislation relating to the precautions to be taken may differ from country to country, but the following examples illustrate the sort of attention that has to be paid to laboratory design and procedure. Regulations for work with category 2 organisms (Hazard Group 2 in the UK; organisms to be studied at Biosafety Level 2 in the USA) include the requirement for sufficient space (24 m^3 per person is recommended), for impervious bench tops so that disinfection can be effected, for all contaminated materials to be decontaminated before disposal, and for staff to be trained in working with pathogens, and to be supervised by a competent scientist. Floors should be easy to clean, preferably having sealed skirtings, and laboratory furniture should either be suspended on legs or be sealed into the floor covering so as to obviate problems arising from spilt cultures being held in cracks or under furniture units. Suitable disinfectants should be available and procedures maintained for renewal of working-strength solutions as appropriate (e.g. 24 hours in the case of diluted hypochlorite). Laboratory coats of an approved type, closed in such a way as to afford protection, should be worn in the laboratory and should not be stored with outdoor clothes. Entry to offices should not be through laboratories.

11.5 Biological safety cabinets

Seldom should it be *necessary* to use a biological safety cabinet in a food microbiology laboratory, except for blending and some other processes that may generate a large amount of aerosol, but there may be occasions on which a worker would wish to use one, to minimize the risk of cross-contamination between samples, for example. A Class II cabinet (*British Standard 5726: 1979*), which has an open front and affords some protection to the work (by a supply of filtered laminar flow of air down on to the work surface) as well as to the worker, would probably be the most useful type to have available. It should be serviced annually and also if it is moved (movement of the cabinet may break seals or crack the filter), and air flow should be monitored regularly. (The numbers used to designate various types of biological safety cabinets in the UK bear no relation to the categories of pathogens; they refer to types of design of the cabinets.)

Several of the moulds and yeasts associated with the spoilage of foods can cause lung infections. Because dispersal of these organisms is naturally achieved through the production and distribution by air currents of vast numbers of low-density spores such as conidia, the food microbiologist would be well advised to use a safety cabinet when culturing them.

11.6 Chemical aspects of laboratory safety

Many chemicals are hazardous to health; some are more hazardous than others. Workers in laboratories should assess *and record* the risk posed by each chemical and every other substance *in the context of its proposed use*. In the UK this requirement is imposed by the *Control of Substances Hazardous to Health Regulations 1988 (COSHH)*. These impose good discipline because they require the worker to know about the hazards posed by the substances with which he or she works and to be aware of any special neutralization and disposal procedures that may be required. Chemical companies must provide hazard data sheets for any chemicals they supply. Several companies also produce books and computer discs of information. However, the information is not always as useful as might initially appear because the companies have to warn about all possibilities and they do not know the type of use to which their products will be put. Therefore one may be warned that sucrose and sodium chloride may be dangerous if ingested and that one has to wash one's hands in soap and water if they get pure water on them! Informed interpretation of the data on chemical safety in the context of proposed use is therefore an important part of assessments, and is not easy. Some ingredients of selective media are hazardous and so considerable caution may be required when weighing powdered media prior to rehydration. Some medical antibiotics pose considerable hazards and so should not be ignored. Ideally, dangerous substances should be purchased as solutions to minimize the risk of particles being released into the atmosphere during weighing and other procedures.

Botulinum toxin, being extremely potent, should not be worked with in a routine food microbiology laboratory. Any suspect material should be autoclaved, although specimens may be transferred to specialist laboratories by approved means. Material containing mycotoxins should be handled with care as several of these toxins are carcinogens and are very resistant to heat. Such materials are biodegradable and so can be put in well-managed tips, providing there is no chance of their entering the food chain; alternatively they have to be incinerated. Work with pure mycotoxins should be undertaken only in highly specialized rooms where extreme care will be taken to avoid contamination of workers and the environment.

11.7 Control of the risk of fire

Flammable solvents should be stored and used with care. All except small quantities should be kept in outside stores or in metal cabinets designed specially for flammable solvents. Such cabinets should be firmly closed except when containers are being removed or replaced. They should not be placed on possible fire exit escape routes. Fire exits should be clearly marked and kept free from combustible material and items which might impede rapid escape. Doors intended to contain fires should not be propped open, unless by stops that automatically close the doors in the event of fire. Flammable solvents should not be stored in refrigerators or freezers unless these are 'sparkproof'.

High concentrations of hydrogen should not be used to achieve an anaerobic atmosphere. It is safer to use a gas mixture of not more than 10 % hydrogen, with 5–10 % carbon dioxide and the remainder of nitrogen, in conjunction with an anaerobic jar or cabinet that has a cold catalyst, or to use a commercially available gas generation pack (but see Section 12.7).

11.8 Laboratory philosophy

Laboratories are places for practical work by skilled professional scientists and technicians. Laboratory coats, stout shoes and often safety spectacles should be worn by all who enter. Maintenance, security, secretarial and other non-laboratory staff should not enter laboratory areas without first reporting to the person in charge of the laboratory, who will decide if it is necessary for them to put on protective clothing. Persons such as senior managers should not feel that they and their visitors can pass freely between laboratory and production areas. Trolleys containing material for autoclaving should not pass through regular passageways for non-technical staff. Recreational and refreshment areas should be provided away from the laboratories, and food and drink for consumption should never be brought to the laboratory. Smoking, eating, drinking and the application of cosmetics should not be allowed in the laboratory. All personnel should be aware that if something does go wrong as a result of failure to follow safe procedures there will be criticism from all quarters. Viewed after an accident, a particular procedure may seem grossly negligent, whereas before it had seemed reasonable; condemnation of individuals deemed negligent may become intense. People have been known to commit suicide in connection with failure to ensure safe procedures at work. In short, laboratories are specialized areas that require careful planning, sufficient resources and rigorous supervision.

11.9 A checklist of some points for the safe functioning of a laboratory

Administration

Who have responsibility for overseeing safety aspects in the laboratory, the department, the building, the company, and do these persons have knowledge of government safety requirements and pass this knowledge to others as appropriate?

Is there a safety committee with representatives of various groups of workers, and does it hold regular meetings with minutes available to all employees?

Are there written safety instructions for work in the laboratory and do all workers receive them?

Are safety notices such as 'Wear safety spectacles' displayed as appropriate, and are they obeyed?

Is there a formal procedure for monitoring proposals to undertake work involving a high fire risk, recognized pathogens, dangerous chemicals or genetic manipulation?

Is entry to the laboratory restricted and monitored?

Are procedures established for the training of newly appointed workers?

Is the responsibility that every person carries for safety clearly recognized by all?

First Aid

Are first-aid boxes available, regularly checked, and the checking recorded?

Is everyone informed about the basics of first aid?

Are registered first aiders available and is their training regularly updated?

Are first-aid notices posted, giving names and telephone numbers of first aiders and others, for use in an emergency?

Are telephones readily available, including for out-of-hours working?

Procedure for out-of-hours working

Is any working alone allowed?

What is the procedure for keeping a note of workers in the building out-of-hours?

General microbiological procedures

Are all microbiological procedures performed under the supervision of an experienced microbiologist who is conversant with government requirements and is responsible for training staff?

Media preparation and wash-up

Are autoclaves checked annually, along with other pressure vessels?

Are dated thermograph records of autoclaves made and kept?

Is the use of autoclaves restricted to trained staff?

Is a sufficient cooling period allowed, after heating under pressure, to avoid boiling on release of pressure?

Do routine procedures ensure that only microbiologically uncontaminated, disinfected or autoclaved items are washed up?

Are all contaminated disposable plastics autoclaved before disposal?

Are hypodermic needles, scalpel blades and other 'sharps' placed in an approved container, autoclaved and, if not rendered safe by melted plastic, incinerated?

General Hygiene

Are laboratory coats of an approved design worn by all persons in the laboratory and are they properly closed?

What is the procedure for laundering of laboratory coats? It may be that autoclaving prior to laundry will be necessary only in the event of an accident.

Is storage of non-work personal belongings, including food for consumption, not allowed in the laboratory?

Are gloves and safety spectacles readily available?

Are hand-washing facilities provided in the laboratory at designated sinks with disinfectant soap?

Are benches wiped down with disinfectant after work and after any accident?

Is there a recognized procedure for dealing with spillages and breakages, and are required disinfectants and receptacles readily available?

Fire precautions

Are there sufficient fire doors and fire exits and are all fire exits and stairwells clearly marked and kept free from debris?

Are fire doors kept closed (or on a system to allow automatic closure in the event of fire)?

Is any lift clearly marked so as not to be used in the event of fire?

Are flammable packages and other materials discarded as soon as they are no longer required?

Are procedures for the safe storage of flammable solvents understood and enforced?

Are fire alarms clearly marked and regularly checked?

Are fire drills held at least twice per year?

Are various types of fire extinguishers readily available, regularly checked, and their use understood by workers?

Is there a list of persons who know the siting of gas cylinders, flammable solvents, etc.?

Are 'What to do in the event of fire' notices displayed?

Centrifuges

Do centrifuge lids have safety locks?

Is there an established procedure for dealing with the escape of microbes from centrifuge tubes and for the safe cleaning of rotors?

Is there a logging and servicing procedure for centrifuges as appropriate?

Are potential users trained in the use of centrifuges – balancing, choice of correct tubes and closures, etc?

Chemicals
Are *all* substances in the laboratory assessed for safety in the context of their use and are the assessments recorded?

Who checks that safety aspects are understood before a chemical is ordered?

Are chemicals stored in a safe manner, with incompatible substances not in close proximity?

Gas cylinders
Are all cylinders clamped in position or on gas cylinder trolleys?

Are their positions known to potential firefighters?

Are they checked with soap solution, etc. to ensure absence of leaks?

Is 10 % hydrogen in nitrogen or in nitrogen plus carbon dioxide used in place of pure hydrogen whenever possible?

Fume cupboards
Do fume cupboards have an adequate air flow, checked by visual monitor on the machine before every use and by an independent flow meter at least twice per year?

Are motors checked and serviced annually?

Are the cupboards sited away from strong air currents and passageways?

Can the cupboards be locked closed when maintenance staff are working on ducts, etc?

Safety cabinets for microbiological work
Are all relevant workers clear about the distinction between biological safety cabinets and laminar flow cabinets of a type designed solely to protect the work (*not the worker*) from contamination?

Do they realize that open-fronted safety cabinets must be sited away from strong air currents because efficiency depends on a steady inflow of air to the cabinet?

Are flow rates checked visually before every use and twice yearly by an independent meter?

Are the cabinets serviced annually, and are they fumigated before servicing?

Are the cabinets checked by a particle-release method every time they are moved or a filter is changed?

Electrical

Are building wiring and sockets checked periodically, including as required by government legislation?

Are electrical cut-off points clearly marked and readily accessible?

Is a fuse with the smallest possible rating used in plugs of all apparatus and is the outer cable of equipment clamped in the plug?

Are leads kept as far as possible away from sinks and water?

Is all apparatus checked annually, and prominently marked as checked?

Radiation

Is it understood that no work with radioactive materials may be undertaken before ensuring that appropriate government requirements are met?

Methods for assessing microbiological quality

This book is not a laboratory manual, so we do not give full details of the methods to be used. These may be found in sources such as the relevant ISO standards, Harrigan & McCance (1976), or ICMSF (1978). The purpose of this chapter is rather to suggest to the reader the way in which the food microbiologist should approach the application of the various recommended methods, always questioning the validity of their application for the uses to which they are being put.

12.1 Standardization of laboratory methods

The International Committee (now known as 'Commission') on Microbiological Specifications for Foods (ICMSF) was formed by the International Association (now 'Union') of Microbiological Societies (IUMS) in 1962. It was formed because of the importance of reaching international agreement on the laboratory methodology to be used in the determination of the conformance or nonconformance of foods to microbiological specifications. It is imperative that a microbiological specification for a food should include a description of the methods (diluent, media, incubation temperature, etc.) to be used, because the choice of method may dramatically affect the result. ICMSF's first book, *Micro-organisms in Foods, Volume I, Their Significance and Methods of Enumeration*, which was published in 1968, had as its aim the eventual international agreement on the appropriate methodology to be adopted for the detection and enumeration of a range of microorganisms and/or their toxins. Nevertheless, in many cases ICMSF described a number of different methods for the detection of a specific organism, and even in the second edition of this book there remain several multiple recommendations. For example, it describes four plating procedures for enumeration of coagulase-positive staphylococci and three Most Probable Number (MPN) procedures for coliforms.

The International Standards Organization publishes recommended standard procedures for various methods for the microbiological examination of foods. These are sometimes the same as, and sometimes different from, ICMSF methods. National standards organizations (e.g. the British Standards Institution)'have also published recommended methods, which may or may not be identical with ISO methods. International commodity groups (e.g. the International Dairy Federation) have also felt it necessary to publish their own recommendations. Many governments incorporate microbiological specifications, with or without analytical methods, into their national legislation.

Thus, there could be a range of possible methods imposed from without upon a food microbiologist working in a Quality Assurance (QA) laboratory. It should be remembered, however, that the food microbiologist should be aiming to maximize the recovery rate of the organisms being enumerated in a particular food. The food environment itself, and the metabolic state of the organisms in that food, may substantially affect the recovery efficiency of a given procedure. In particular, the choice of diluent (or the incorporation of a pre-treatment procedure) and the choice of a resuscitation technique may need to be validated in relation to the specific food or the specific production process. It is difficult to incorporate such a degree of flexibility into published specifications, standards or statutory procedures.

In the following sections some examples are provided of the extensive range of recommended procedures to be found in the references given in the bibliography, and of the possible shortcomings of these procedures.

12.2 Preparation of dilutions

Since the decimal dilution series is nearly always prepared volumetrically by pipette, it is preferable to prepare the first 10^{-1} dilution by, for example, weighing out 10 g of food, suspending or homogenizing the food in an appropriate diluent, transferring this mixture to a container marked at 100 ml, and making up to volume with diluent. Then counts can be calculated per gram of food with reasonable accuracy, since 1 ml of this mixture will contain 0.1 g of food. The often-used method (ICMSF, 1978) of preparing a 10^{-1} dilution by adding 90 ml of diluent to 10 g of food and preparing subsequent dilutions volumetrically introduces an uncertainty into the calculation as the extent of solubility of the food is unknown.

A 0.1 % peptone solution at pH 6.8–7.0 is a commonly used diluent (ICMSF, 1978). However, 0.1 % peptone + 0.85 % sodium chloride has been specified in *ISO 6887*; the equivalent British Standard (*BS 5763: Part 6*) also comments that this diluent should be used 'unless there is evidence that other diluents are better suited'.

The possible modification of the nature of the diluent by the sample at the lowest dilution (i.e. highest concentration) should not be overlooked. In particular, if the food sample contains a high proportion of undissolved water-soluble material (e.g. as in the case of milk powders, dehydrated soups, crisp flavourings) what will be the effect of its solution in the diluent? Will the pH or a_w be greatly affected? If in doubt the pH of the first dilution should be checked, and a_w can be checked using an appropriate instrument (e.g. a SINA equi-hygroscope or Protimeter). If there has been a pH change, the method will need to be modified to incorporate a pH buffer into the diluent. If the food has a high content of undissolved soluble solids, and hence a low a_w, a diluent with a lower concentration of solutes may be chosen to allow for this.

Certain microbiological assessments may call for special diluents. For example, to avoid damage by oxygen when examining for anaerobes, Reinforced Clostridial Medium (RCM) or a similar medium may be used to maintain a low redox potential and the sample may be dispersed in the diluent by a method that minimizes incorporation of oxygen into the mixture – a Colworth Stomacher is better than either a top-drive homogenizer or a bottom-drive blender, unless the sample container is flushed with oxygen-free nitrogen before blending. When culturing very oxygen-sensitive anaerobes, an anaerobic work station should be used.

Sterile 20 % sucrose solution, or 15 % sodium chloride solution can be used when examining foods of low a_w for the presence respectively of osmotolerant microbes or extreme halophiles capable of growing at low a_w, to avoid osmotic shock.

12.3 Aerobic mesophilic counts

It is most important to emphasize that there is no cultural method for determining the 'total viable count' of a mixed microflora of unknown composition as is found in most foods. The choice of medium, incubation temperature and gaseous atmosphere will tend to allow the growth of some organisms and not to allow the growth of others. Obviously, therefore, an Aerobic Mesophilic Count (AMC) should *never* be referred to as a 'Total Viable Count'. It cannot even represent a total aerobic mesophilic count, because of the effect of the choice of medium, temperature and time.

Furthermore, it must not be assumed that a colony always derives from only a single organism. Bacteria may occur as clumps or chains which may not become fragmented on dilution. Thus it is more correct to refer to a viable count in terms of colony-forming units per gram (c.f.u. g^{-1}) rather than bacteria per gram.

The AMC (which may also be known as a Standard Plate Count) does not necessarily correlate with food safety – many pathogens would not grow under the cultural conditions used. However, it is often used as an indicator of the general standard of hygiene and of temperature control in the food premises, and during distribution and storage of the food.

The standard medium of choice is Glucose Tryptone Yeast Extract Agar (also known as Plate Count Agar; PCA; and Standard Methods Agar), with incubation at 30°C (*ISO 4833*; ICMSF 1978).

If the interest is in the spoilage potential of the microflora, then the chosen medium should simulate the habitat, or at least contain the same range of nutrients as the food in question. For example, for an AMC on dairy products, PCA + 0.1 % skimmed milk has been suggested (*BS 4285*).

12.4 Indicator and index organisms

The term 'indicator organisms' can be applied to any taxonomic, physiological or ecological group of organisms whose presence or absence provides indirect evidence concerning a particular feature in the past history of the sample. It is often associated with organisms of intestinal origin but other groups may act as indicators for other situations. For example, the presence of members of the set 'all Gram-negative bacteria' in heat-treated foodstuffs is indicative of inadequate heat-treatment (relative to the initial numbers of these organisms) or of contamination subsequent to heating. Coliform counts, since coliforms represent only a sub-set of 'all Gram-negative bacteria', provide a much less sensitive indicator of problems associated with heat treatment, but are still frequently used in the examination of heat-treated foodstuffs. (Harrigan & McCance, 1976)

The term 'index organism' was suggested by Ingram in 1977 (Mossel, 1982) for a marker whose presence indicated the possible presence of an ecologically similar pathogen.

12.4.1 Enterobacteriaceae

ICMSF (1978) and *ISO 7402* concur in recommending the use of Crystal Violet Neutral Red Bile Glucose Agar (VRBGA) incubated at 35–37°C for colony counts of the *Enterobacteriaceae*. When small numbers are suspected, an MPN count can be used; *ISO 7402* recommends the use of Buffered Brilliant Green Bile Glucose Broth at 35–37°C for 24 hours, with subculture from each tube on to VRBGA.

12.4.2 Coliform counts

ICMSF (1978) and *ISO 4832* agree on the use of Crystal Violet Neutral Red Bile Lactose Agar (VRBA), but the former recommended incubation at 30 ± 1°C for 24 ± 2 hours, whereas the latter specifies 35–37°C for the same period. It is obvious that there is a high probability of the non-equivalence of these two methods with many food types, since there may be present saprophytic lactose-fermenting members of the *Enterobacteriaceae* unable to grow (or unable to ferment lactose) at the higher temperatures.

In the case of MPN counts there is also a lack of agreement. *ISO 4831* specifies Brilliant Green Bile Lactose Broth (BGLB) incubated at 30 ± 1°C, whereas ICMSF (1978) listed three different media, all incubated at 35–37°C: the 'British' method, using MacConkey's broth; the 'North American' method using Lauryl Sulphate Tryptose Broth subcultured into BGLB; and BGLB subcultured on to VRBA or Endo Agar. Once again, the non-equivalence of these methods is obvious.

12.4.3 Escherichia coli

In the case of *E. coli*, the ICMSF (1978) and ISO methods are somewhat different from one another; since *E. coli* is a true taxonomic group the non-equivalence of the methods is frequently overlooked. For example, *ISO 7251* specifies a modified Eijkman test being carried out using EC Broth, incubated at $45 \pm 0.5°C$, whereas ICMSF (1978) recommended EC Broth incubated at $44.5 \pm 0.2°C$ (N. American method) or BGLB incubated at $44 \pm 0.1°C$ (European method). This elevated temperature is being used to eliminate those 'coliforms' which are more sensitive to high temperatures than is *E. coli*, so it is obvious that small differences in the incubation temperature will profoundly affect the growth response of organisms when that temperature is around the maximum for their growth. Many water-baths today have electronic controllers that give temperatures to within ± 0.1 or even $\pm 0.05°C$, so the temperature differences in combination with different media of possibly different selectivity in these recommended methods can be significant.

12.5 Detection and enumeration of pathogenic and toxigenic organisms

The laboratory procedures for assessing the hazard of a food-poisoning syndrome caused by ingestion of viable organisms (Chapter 4), have traditionally depended on the use of highly selective media. Very often, assessment of a hazard from toxigenic organisms (e.g. *Staphylococcus aureus*) (Chapter 3) is based similarly on the use of selective media to detect the viable organisms, although the syndrome is caused by ingestion of a preformed toxin which may be present in the food even when a process has subsequently rendered the causative organisms non-viable. As the toxins involved become chemically and serologically characterized, detection techniques based upon these characters become available (e.g. aflatoxin can be detected by TLC, HPLC or ELISA, staphylococcal enterotoxin can be detected by ELISA).

Many of the isolation techniques of conventional microbiology recommended for the detection of pathogens or toxigenic organisms include liquid-enrichment procedures capable of detecting low concentrations of organisms (Harrigan & McCance, 1976; ICMSF, 1978). The stages in isolation and identification can be generalized as:

(1) pretreatment of the sample if necessary (e.g. concentration, centrifugation);

(2) resuscitation in a 'non-selective' medium;

(3) selective enrichment in a liquid medium;

(4) detection on solid selective and/or differential media;

(5) purification of isolates on a non-selective, differential medium;

(6) confirmatory biochemical, physiological and other tests;

(7) typing by serology, bacteriophage, etc. if appropriate.

The full procedure may take up to 2 weeks to complete, but this may be shortened by the use of rapid alternative procedures to bypass some of the stages. These possibilities will be discussed in Chapter 13.

It is better to combine a liquid-enrichment stage and a solid selective stage which use different selective agents, since otherwise the second stage is unlikely to provide any further selection against unwanted organisms. For example, if, in attempting to detect small numbers of *S. aureus*, Giolitti & Cantoni's tellurite-containing liquid enrichment medium be followed by Baird-Parker's tellurite-containing medium, any tellurite-tolerant organisms which are *not S. aureus* will grow in the first medium, and then will not be selected against by the solid medium.

ISO and ICMSF have recommended a range of standardized detection and isolation procedures for many commonly sought organisms. Notwithstanding this, it should be remembered that the effectiveness of a given enrichment or selective isolation (in terms of both sensitivity to low concentrations of all strains of the target organisms and selectivity against other interfering microflorae) may depend as much on the unintentional modification of the medium caused by the addition of (usually) appreciable amounts of food as it does upon the recipe used to prepare the medium. Obviously, different foods will have different effects on different media. A possible approach to the standardization of detection methods is to specify for each pathogen the resuscitation stage and first liquid-enrichment stage appropriate for the particular food being examined, with later stages then being common to the examination of all categories of sample. Because of the time taken to investigate and validate such food-specific methods, the specification of these first steps has been attempted by institutions such as ICMSF, ISO, AOAC for only a very few foods and a very few organisms (e.g.

Salmonella in dried, frozen, or heat-treated foods). It therefore behoves workers to consider carefully the types of questions mentioned in Section 12.2.

12.6 Enteric pathogenic E. coli

From the point of view of selective isolation using selective, differential media, we can distinguish two groups: the rapid fermenters of lactose, and those that ferment lactose slowly or not at all.

12.6.1 The rapid fermenters of lactose
These can be detected and counted using techniques similar to those adopted for normal counts of *E. coli*, followed by serotyping or by detection of the toxins by ELISA, etc. (Chapter 13). To apply serological typing to all isolates of *E. coli* would however be expensive and time-consuming.

Attention must be paid to the physiological and growth characteristics of some of the pathogenic strains. More specific detection and isolation procedures for the pathogenic strains, including techniques for detecting particular serovars such as 0157:H7, are being developed; these may incorporate immunodiagnostic assays such as ELISA, or nucleic acid probe methods within, or on, the primary detection or counting step (Chapter 13).

The verocytotoxic *E. coli* (VTEC), the predominant serovars of which are 0157:H7 and 0157:H−, are not detected successfully by growth techniques employing elevated incubation temperatures around 44–45°C. These organisms are sorbitol-negative, whereas most *E. coli* strains are sorbitol-positive, so VTEC 0157 can be isolated using a MacConkey's agar incorporating 1 % D-sorbitol instead of lactose, incubated for 24 hours at 37°C (see also PHLS 1990a, b). Note also that these organisms give a negative result in the 4-methylumbelliferone glucuronide fluorogenic assay technique which is used by many workers as a quick screening and counting method for *E. coli*.

12.6.2 Lactose-negative and slow-fermenting strains of E. coli
These include the EIEC strains (see Chapter 4). We should consider *Shigella* here, rather than under Section 12.7, since firstly there is much evidence that shigellae do not enrich and grow well in the conditions tolerated by salmonellae, and secondly it is as well not to confuse these organisms with the (possibly rare) slow lactose-fermenting salmonellae that have been reported. ICMSF (1978) suggested using nutrient broth pre-enrichment, followed by selective enrichment in

Mossel's brilliant green glucose ox-gall broth (EE broth), with isolation on MacConkey agar. It is suggested alternatively that the selective enrichment and isolation of shigellae should be by use of Hajna's GN broth and Taylor's XLD agar respectively.

12.7 *Salmonella*

Salmonella will often have suffered some injury in foods as a result of various processing procedures such as heating, drying, freezing. Whereas growing cells of *Salmonella* may be tolerant of Selenite Broth or Tetrathionate Broth, it is highly likely that metabolically injured salmonellae will not recover in these enrichment media. Consequently, most standard procedures have accommodated this problem by recommending resuscitation in a 'non-selective' medium such as Buffered Peptone Water before sub-culturing into the selective enrichment medium. *ISO 6579* specifies resuscitation (often called a 'pre-enrichment' stage) in Buffered Peptone Water, but ICMSF (1978) listed seven possible pre-enrichment media, choice depending on the nature of the food commodity being examined. In some cases the 'medium' sounds a little surprising – for example, Distilled Water or Distilled Water + 20 p.p.m. Brilliant Green, but such an initial stage would be indicated especially for dried foodstuffs with a high soluble solids content. Silverstolpe *et al.* (1961) reported an outbreak of *Salmonella muenchen* food poisoning amongst infants which was caused by a dried baby feed. They discovered that the preferred diluent was distilled water, since normal media resulted in a mixture with a bacteriostatically or bactericidally low a_w.

This stage is followed by two selective enrichment procedures run in tandem: Selenite Cystine Broth at 35 or 37°C, *and* either Tetrathionate Broth at 43°C (*ISO 6579*) or Tetrathionate Brilliant Green Broth at 43°C (ICMSF, 1978).

The next stage, using solid selective, differential media also shows a divergence between ISO and ICMSF. *ISO 6579* specifies Brilliant Green Phenol Red Agar (BGPRA) *and* a second medium of the laboratory's choice. ICMSF recommended BGPRA *and* Wilson & Blair's Bismuth Sulphite Agar *and* a third medium of the laboratory's choice. Since various serovars of *Salmonella* show different sensitivities to these selective media, this will be a crucial stage in the isolation technique.

Both procedures include the use of Triple Sugar Iron Agar (TSI) in the confirmatory biochemical tests. It is important to be careful in the interpretation of this screening procedure. In the USA, food-poisoning outbreaks caused by lactose-fermenting salmonellae have been reported. Obviously a procedure that discards lactose-positive organisms is unable to determine whether lactose-fermenting salmonellae are common, rare, or even non-existent! Consequently, this led to the AOAC recommending that both lactose-negative *and* lactose-positive isolates should be examined by serology.

12.8 *Clostridium perfringens*

Angelotti's sulphite polymyxin sulphadiazine agar has been widely used in the past (see Harrigan & McCance, 1976), but some strains of *Clostridium perfringens* are inhibited by this medium, so ICMSF (1978) recommended the use of either Harmon's egg-yolk sulphite cycloserine agar or Shahidi & Ferguson's egg-yolk polymyxin kanamycin sulphite agar. In the UK Public Health Laboratory Service there has been a long tradition of using neomycin blood agar as the isolation medium; however, although this seems to work well when detecting the large numbers of *C. perfringens* found in a food that has caused an outbreak of *C. perfringens* food poisoning or in the faeces of the patients, this medium does not seem to be sufficiently selective to be used in quality assurance in the food industry where the medium has to cope with detecting smaller numbers of the organism when they may be masked by much larger numbers of other organisms in a food material. The use of egg-yolk-free tryptose sulphite cycloserine agar is specified by *ISO 7937*.

The plates must be incubated anaerobically. This is normally achieved by using an anaerobic jar, although if many anaerobic counts are being performed at the same time, an anaerobic incubator may be more practicable.

A number of different methods can be used to obtain the anaerobic atmosphere (see Harrigan & McCance, 1976). These can involve the use of a cylinder of oxygen-free nitrogen, a nitrogen/hydrogen mixture, or hydrogen; a chemical source of hydrogen external to the jar (but consider safety, Section 11.7) or the use of a disposable hydrogen-generating envelope placed in the anaerobic jar. In all cases there should be supplementation with carbon dioxide. These different techniques will give rise to different oxygen-free atmospheres which are predominantly nitrogen, or nitrogen/hydrogen mixtures, or predominantly hydrogen, with carbon dioxide. It has usually been assumed that all these methods are interchangeable (e.g. see Pierson & Stern, 1986) and have no effect on the recoverability of *C. perfringens*, but it would appear that such conclusions have often been drawn from pure culture work which has examined normal unstressed bacterial cultures. There is evidence that *C. perfringens* spores which have been damaged by heat, for example in heat-treated or dried foods, may show different recovery rates in the different anaerobic atmospheres (probably because of the different equilibrium redox potentials that will result in the isolation media; Futter & Richardson, 1971). Until this question has been properly resolved, it would be as well to validate the procedure to be adopted by comparing the recovery rates of the different methods of obtaining anaerobiosis in respect of the particular foods or food processing procedures under investigation.

12.9 *Bacillus cereus*

Colony counts of presumptive *B. cereus* may be obtained using either Mossel's Mannitol Egg-yolk Phenol-red Polymyxin Agar (MEPP) or Holbrook & Anderson's Polymyxin Pyruvate Egg-yolk Mannitol Bromothymol Blue Agar (PPEMB), incubated at 35–37°C for 24 hours. The differential characteristics of these media depend on lecithinase production by *B. cereus* and the *non*-fermentation of mannitol by *B. cereus*. Since the media are not well buffered, and some other species of *Bacillus* possess a lecithinase, care should be taken not to incubate the plates for too long, as otherwise growth of mannitol-fermenting organisms may mask the lack of fermentation by *B. cereus* colonies.

This short incubation period leads the food microbiologist into a dilemma, since bacterial *spores* may take a considerable time to germinate – one study revealed a log-normal distribution for germination with many of the viable spores present germinating after more than 2 weeks. In any microbiological examination of foods for bacterial spores, whether *C. perfringens*, *B. cereus* or other organism, quite frequently the ratio of spores to vegetative cells will be high, and in some processed foods (e.g. heat-treated or dried foods) vegetative cells may be rare or absent. This contrasts with the situation found by the public-health microbiologist examining foods suspected of having caused an outbreak, or faecal specimens of patients, in both of which vegetative organisms can be expected in large numbers.

It is to be hoped that commercially available ELISA or other diagnostic kits will soon enable the direct detection of *B. cereus* enterotoxins in foods.

12.10 *Staphylococcus aureus*

As with *B. cereus*, the food microbiologist is interested in both the viable organisms and the enterotoxin. Since the staphylococcal enterotoxin is much more heat-resistant than the bacteria, dried foods (e.g. dried milk) may contain clinically significant amounts of the enterotoxin whilst viable bacteria are not detectable.

12.10.1 *Detection of the organisms*

A number of different media are currently in use, and ICMSF (1978) listed five recommended methods of enumeration. Most solid media incorporate tellurium salts as a primary selective agent, some use sodium chloride instead. Similarly, liquid selective enrichment broths used to detect low concentrations may contain either tellurite or sodium chloride. In general, it is preferable not to use the sodium chloride-containing media on foods containing appreciable amounts of salt since all microorganisms growing on such foods will be salt-tolerant.

Usually, *S. aureus* will be confirmed by checking on such characteristics as coagulase production or thermostable nuclease production and then assuming that such organisms are probably capable of producing enterotoxins, rather than looking directly for enterotoxigenicity, primarily because at present the kits available for detecting enterotoxins are seen as being rather expensive.

12.10.2 *Staphylococcal enterotoxins*

ICMSF (1978) recommended two methods of extracting and concentrating enterotoxin from foods, followed by detection and identification by the microslide gel immunodiffusion test. The microgram sensitivity of these techniques is not sufficient to detect the minimum (nanogram) concentration of enterotoxin in foods which can cause the clinical syndrome when consumed by sensitive individuals. The ELISA technique enables nanogram quantities to be detected.

12.11 *Listeria monocytogenes*

Since the increased interest in the rôle of food as a cause of human listeriosis, there has been much developmental work on media for the selective isolation of *L. monocytogenes*. The most effective combination of liquid selective enrichment and solid selective medium seems to be the use of an Acriflavine Cycloheximide Nalidixic Acid Enrichment Broth, followed by plating on to Oxford Agar (this agar medium contains a 'cocktail' of selective inhibitors). It has been found that some listeriae are rather acriflavine-sensitive on first isolation from foods, so a double enrichment procedure is often used, with the first liquid enrichment employing a rather low concentration of acriflavine (12 p.p.m.), and the secondary liquid enrichment incorporating double the concentration of acriflavine (25 p.p.m.). The species are differentiated by biochemical tests, and *L. monocytogenes* distinguished from the others by the CAMP test for synergistic haemolysis.

12.12 *Campylobacter* spp.

Campylobacters were not widely recognized as causes of intestinal disease before 1977, although there is good reason to suppose that they have been responsible for much foodborne enteritis over many years. Detection requires specialized techniques – selective filtration, utilizing the ability of campylobacters but of few other bacteria to pass through 0.45 µm or 0.65 µm membrane filters, or selection by the use of a combination of several antimicrobial agents. Plates of a nutritionally rich medium should be incubated in an atmosphere containing 5 % oxygen and 10 % carbon dioxide. This can be obtained by either using a cylinder containing an appropriate gas mixture to replace some air in an anaerobic jar, or gas-generating envelopes designed specifically for culture of *Campylobacter*. Thus campylobacters provide a good example of how the assessment of the safety of a food is utterly dependent on the efficacy of the detection procedures used.

12.13 *Vibrio parahaemolyticus*

Selective enrichment of most vibrios may be achieved by using alkaline peptone water containing 1 % sodium chloride, incubated at 37°C for only 5–8 hours, or at 20°C overnight. The incubation period is critical, since the pH will drop during incubation, and then other organisms will be able to overgrow the vibrios. In addition, it should be noted that modification of the pH of the medium may occur as a result of addition of the food sample. For this reason, selective enrichment media such as Salt Colistin Broth or Glucose Salt Teepol Broth, which are *not* dependent on high pH, are more usually employed in food microbiology. A commonly used solid selective medium (readily obtainable from manufacturers of dehydrated and ready-prepared media) is Thiosulphate Citrate Bile Salt Sucrose Agar, incubated at 37°C.

12.14 *Yersinia enterocolitica*

Yersinia enterocolitica can be isolated using the typical selective principles for the *Enterobacteriaceae*, such as media containing bile salts or brilliant green. Since the organism is psychrotrophic, a medium such as MacConkey agar can be made selective for *Y. enterocolitica* by incubation at 4°C. Similarly, liquid enrichment can be achieved by using media such as Enterobacteriaceae Enrichment Broth incubated at 4°C. Obviously, the incubation period must be extended at this low temperature, and incubation periods of 3–6 weeks are used with care being taken to prevent evaporation of water from the medium.

The usual procedure is to employ cold selection only at the liquid-enrichment stage, incubating for 3 weeks at 4°C. Each week the broth is streaked on to a solid selective medium. A medium that has been developed specifically for *Y. enterocolitica* is Schiemann's Cefsulodin Irgasan Novobiocin Agar (available from many suppliers of dehydrated and ready-prepared media). Plates are incubated at 32°C.

13

Rapid methods for assessing microbiological quality

13.1 The need for rapid methods

It is becoming increasingly recognized that food poisoning and foodborne diseases are very common and that both these public health problems and the microbiological spoilage of foods can be minimized by the careful choice of raw materials and correct manufacturing and storage procedures. Achievement of such objectives requires, in many cases, monitoring at various stages to assess the total microbiological load or to look for particular types. Because such procedures using traditional methods are labour intensive and often take considerable time before results are available, a great deal of effort has gone into developing rapid methods, and producing apparatus and reagents to overcome these disadvantages. In this chapter we will outline the principles of some of these methods and discuss some of their advantages and disadvantages.

13.2 Methods for assessing general microbiological load

Five types of procedure have been developed: those that produce colony counts more rapidly than traditional methods; those that rely on direct detection of microbes by microscopy; those that assess the amount of some particular component of microbes and assume the value obtained is proportional to numbers; those that exploit some physiological property of the organisms; and those that assay products of metabolism. We will consider examples of some of these methods.

13.2.1 Speeding the colony count procedure

Improvements in homogenization techniques (mainly by use of the Colworth Stomacher), developments in dilution procedures (by use of automatic pipettes accurately delivering small quantities, and the Spiral Systems spiral plater, which achieves a wide range of dilutions over a single plate), and application of automatic image analysers for counting colonies have all helped to update the traditional colony-counting technique for estimating microbial load. Simple ideas to save time have been developed and found several applications. The agar slide, provided sterile in a container, is dipped into a liquid sample and so inoculated with approximately a standard volume, or pressed on a surface, and then incubated in its original container to give a rapid estimate of the range of organisms present. The agar sausage can be pressed on a surface to be examined and then a slice removed and placed for incubation until colonies can be counted. All these methods depend on an appropriate medium and set of growth conditions being chosen for the organisms present in the sample, but they have the advantage of linking in with long-established standards for particular foods or ingredients. In most cases, though, they save time in setting up the counts but do not substantially reduce the incubation period necessary before a result is obtained.

13.2.2 Direct enumeration by microscopy

The Breed Smear and membrane filtration total counting methods have been used for many years. The main improvement recently in methods for obtaining direct counts has been achieved by the bringing together of several procedures to give the Direct Epifluorescent Filter Technique (DEFT). The technique has found particular utility in the examination of milk. A sample is filtered through a membrane filter, which will retain all the bacteria, moulds and yeasts present. A fluorescent dye is then applied to stain the microbes and excess washed through the filter. Examination is then undertaken using a microscope which provides illumination with ultraviolet light passed down on to the specimen from above the objective lens. Microbes show as fluorescent particles against a black background. In certain conditions and with the use of appropriate dyes distinction can be made between live and dead organisms. It is possible to couple the microscope to an image analyser to obtain counts automatically.

Another method, which is in the developmental stage, is flow cytometry. A fine jet of suspension is passed through a laser beam and the presence of organisms recorded, the use of differential stains or other marking procedure allowing counts of specific components of the flora to be made. This method seems to have similar limitations in food microbiology to the Coulter electronic particle counter in that non-microbial particulate matter of similar size to microorganisms may be recorded as microorganisms.

13.2.3 Assessment of microbial load by using specific cellular components

13.2.3.1 Estimation of adenosine triphosphate
Adenosine triphosphate (ATP) is a component of the living cells of all organisms which is involved in energy transfer. One of the properties of ATP is that, when it is brought into contact with luciferin and luciferase from the firefly, it will cause the emission of a flash of light. In the presence of excess luciferin and luciferase the flash is proportional to the amount of ATP added. To assess the amount of living biomass in a pure culture of bacteria one extracts the ATP, injects it into a lightproof instrument containing the firefly reagents and a photocell. The amount of light detected is recorded and compared with a standard produced using known amounts of ATP. One assumes that ATP constitutes 0.4 % of the bacterial dry weight and so arrives at a value for the biomass present. The test takes only a few minutes but problems can arise if the suspending medium contains something that interferes with the firefly reaction. Determination of the microbial load of foods is less simple because many foods will themselves contain ATP. One therefore has to use some system for obtaining a value for just the microbial ATP.

13.2.3.2 Estimation of lipopolysaccharide
The lipopolysaccharide (LPS) that is present in the outer membrane of Gram-negative bacteria reacts specifically with the amoebocytes in the haemolymph that bathes the internal tissues of *Limulus*, the horseshoe crab; use is made of this reaction in a specific assay for Gram-negative bacteria. It does not distinguish between live and dead organisms – in fact it will react in a similar manner with isolated LPS.

Dilutions of a suspension of sample are made and the end point determined as the highest dilution that will agglutinate the amoebocytes in the haemolymph. Alternatively a procedure that gives a colour reaction can be used. The method can detect as little as 3×10^{-11}g, fewer than 10 000 bacteria. Such a procedure can be useful for rapid assessment of the amount of Gram-negative bacteria in a sample or as a screening procedure to help decide if there are sufficient Gram-negative bacteria present in a sample to justify a more detailed examination for large numbers of a particular type.

Methods that assess the amount of other cellular components such as DNA, total nucleic acids, and murein components have been used experimentally but have not found a major commercial outlet.

13.2.4 Use of physiological properties to assess microbial load

Dye reduction tests have long been used as rapid tests, particularly in the dairy industry, for assessing microbial load. Several other physiological properties associated with the growth of microbes have been utilized to provide commercially available techniques for largely automated methods for assessment of microbial load. Perhaps the least widely used of these involves microcalorimetry – the amount of heat evolved by organisms in a sample being proportional to the number present.

Measurement of the uptake of a radiolabelled compound, or more commonly of its metabolism to produce radiolabelled carbon dioxide, which is released and assayed, has been developed for some purposes but on safety grounds it is less popular than electrical methods in the food industry.

13.2.4.1 Impedance/conductance methods

Impedance/conductance methods are the most widely used of those based on physiological properties. They involve detection of the change in the electrical properties of a growth medium as microbes grow. Metabolism of the complex molecules of the medium leads to a big increase of small ions, which facilitate the passage of an alternating current. Food samples are added to a suitable medium in a special tube containing electrodes, which is then incubated with the electrodes connected to a monitor. Electrical properties are regularly recorded and if impedance gets sufficiently low (conductance gets sufficiently high) within a preset time the food is judged to be too contaminated. In effect the machine is measuring the time taken for an inoculum to reduce the impedance to a predetermined level, a value which, all other things being equal, will be inversely proportional to the $\log_2$ of the number of bacteria in the inoculum. Such machines (Bactometer, Malthus, Rabit) may be linked to warning systems, valves, etc. to stop production automatically as soon as a faulty sample has shown itself, but detection times are too long for electronic feedback procedures usefully to be applied in most situations in the food industry. Although there are some difficulties with these systems under certain circumstances, for example the medium chosen might not be suitable to allow a particular organism of importance to register its presence, difficulties are being overcome. A cell for trapping and assay of carbon dioxide from organisms such as yeast, which hitherto have been difficult to detect by electrical changes, is now available. The machines are very popular and are used successfully for an increasingly wide range of applications.

13.2.5 Use of metabolites to assess microbial quality

Determining the amount of particular and distinctive products of microbial metabolism in a food can be used in quality assessment. Some examples are: fluorescence for aflatoxins; serological methods, particularly ELISA, for aflatoxins and various bacterial toxins; titratable acidity to assess quality of raw milk or the efficiency of starter bacteria; analysis of headspace gases in blown cans; and diacetyl in citrus juices.

13.3 Rapid methods for the detection of specific types of microorganism

The requirement to detect one and only one type of microbe taxes the ingenuity, but to this is added the requirement to do this quickly, so that products can be cleared for sale without being held up for several days awaiting the results of traditional microbiological tests.

13.3.1 Modern versions of enrichment and selective procedures

The traditional stratagem used to detect a particular kind of microbe in a sample has been to inoculate the sample into, or on, a growth medium that contains nutrients well suited to the required organism, and chemicals to inhibit any other organisms that might also be present. Often, incubation conditions for the medium are also chosen so as to be selective by, for example, use of a high or low temperature or specific gaseous conditions. This approach continues to be valid, and various manufacturers market selective media for particular microbes, sometimes using increasingly sophisticated additional 'tricks' to pick out the required organism. The Oxoid Salmonella Rapid Test is a good example. A sample from food or other material, after incubation in a non-selective medium to increase the number of organisms present, is placed in a growth medium in a jar. Also in the jar are two tubes, each containing at the end in the growth medium a different selective medium and above this an indicator medium. *Salmonella* bacteria can enter the tubes from the growth medium, uninhibited by the selective agents and migrate to the upper indicators, which will change colour in a distinctive manner because of the reactions caused by the physiological characteristics of *Salmonella*. Use of the kit requires little staff time and may give a presumptive positive result within 2 days from receipt of sample.

13.3.2 Impedance/conductance methods using selective media

Another method utilizing selective media involves placing the sample in an appropriate selective medium in a Malthus, Bactometer or Rabit machine to detect changes in the electrical characteristics of the medium if the organism of interest grows.

13.3.3 Detection of chemicals possessed by only the required organism

In contrast to techniques that exploit differences in physiology between the required and other organisms there is a variety of methods which use properties that do not depend on growth characteristics but on some inherent chemical feature possessed by only the required organisms. Such chemical differences may be detected on the surface of the organisms, for example, differences in the lipopolysaccharide on the outer layers of the cell, or in the DNA or RNA of the organisms. Unfortunately, although such tests can usually be performed quickly if a large number of the required organisms are present, it is almost invariably the case in the food industry that one is trying to detect very small numbers of the organisms. Therefore almost all these techniques require incubation of the sample first in an appropriate medium to increase the numbers of required organism sufficiently to provide enough material for the test.

13.3.3.1 The use of antibodies

The use of antibodies that will react with the required organisms but no others forms the basis of many techniques. The antibodies may be polyclonal, that is, produced in the normal way in an animal in response to the injection of an appropriate preparation of the required organisms or their parts; or monoclonal, which involves the cultivation *in vitro* of antibody-producing cells from an injected animal that have been fused with myeloma (cancerous) cells to allow indefinite reproduction and the establishment of a hybrid cell line to produce only one, relevant, antibody. The antibodies may form the basis of an enzyme-linked immunosorbent assay (ELISA), in which the presence of the required organisms is detected by a colour change brought about by an enzyme linked to the antibody. Alternatively, the antibody may be attached to small latex beads which in suspension look like milk. In the presence of the required organisms the beads clump because the organisms are binding them together by interacting with the antibody to form granules. Beads of different specificities that are coloured differently are supplied mixed together in some commercial kits, so that the colour of any clumps that develop differentiates between the serological groups tested for, allowing several tests with one application of reagent.

13.3.3.2 Nucleic acid probes

Any inherent differences between microbes are a reflection of differences in the genetic code. If one wishes to use nucleic acid technology to detect only *Salmonella* bacteria, but all *Salmonella* bacteria, in the presence of other microbes, one has to make use of a particular sequence or sequences of nucleic acid bases that are possessed by *Salmonella* but not by other organisms. This requirement is a difficult one but has been met in some cases. One then prepares a probe, that is, a sample of nucleic acid in single-stranded form corresponding to the relevant portion of single-stranded DNA, which has been labelled in some way, usually with radioactive phosphorus. After appropriate treatment of the sample, usually after incubation to increase numbers, the nucleic acid of the organisms is exposed to the probe. It binds to (that is, it forms a double strand with) only the nucleic acid corresponding sufficiently closely to that of the type of organism required and can be detected after incubation with a photographic plate.

The polymerase chain reaction (PCR) may come to play an important part in various aspects of diagnostic microbiology. Using this procedure it is possible in a very short time to increase exponentially the amount of a particular sequence of DNA without increasing other DNA. After allowing several cycles of reaction to proceed the resultant mix of unconcentrated DNA and the concentrated relevant DNA can be exposed to the probe and detected as before. It is possible, without any prior cultivation in order to increase numbers, to detect DNA from very few of the required microbes in the presence of many millions of other microbes. Although a biochemical method, it is at least as vulnerable to interference by microbial contamination as are traditional microbiological methods.

13.3.3.3 Detection by using genetically engineered bacteriophage

Bacteriophages have long been known to be specific for particular host bacteria. They are specific partly because they require surface structures, that are present on only certain particular bacteria, to facilitate attachment. Use of bacteriophages has long been of value in identifying particular types of bacteria involved in outbreaks of typhoid, other salmonellae and *Staphylococcus aureus*. Now workers are using this facility of a bacteriophage to attack only the type of bacterium of interest to form the basis of a rapid and simple test. Into an infective but non-lethal bacteriophage is inserted, by genetic engineering, the ability to cause an attacked bacterium to luminesce. When a sample containing the organisms of interest is incubated in a suitable medium with such a bacteriophage, the bacteriophage attacks the relevant organisms and gives them the ability to generate light. Luminescence then develops in the medium, indicating that the organisms were present in the original sample.

14
The application of microbiological specifications

As already pointed out, absolute protection against the consumer receiving a defective product cannot be provided except by 100 % inspection. In *inspection by attributes* each item will either conform to a stated specification or will fail to conform, the non-conforming items being defined as *defectives*.

When the sampling and inspection is for the acceptance or rejection of a batch or lot of product, the decision on acceptance or rejection will usually depend on the number of defectives c detected in a sample of n items. A comparison of proposed sampling plans can be made by calculating the probabilities of acceptance for a number of assumed percentage defectives in the product sampled.

Microbiological and compositional specifications are often thought by the general public to relate to the quality of finished food products. However, specifications can also be applied to raw (or processed) materials being brought into a food factory for further processing or for incorporation into a food product. Thus, one company's 'end product' may be another company's 'starting material'. The two companies may agree on a specification – the first company's 'end-product specification', the second company's 'buying specification'.

Acceptance sampling (Section 9.6) represents one of the major fields of statistical quality assurance. For example, a company which receives a shipment of goods (e.g. a raw food for processing) may sample the shipment and then either accept it because it meets the specification, or reject it. Rejection may lead to return of the shipment, or to a price penalty for a batch of below-standard material, with perhaps diversion of the material for other purposes. A company may also apply acceptance sampling to its own activities at various stages of production. A government agency or port authority may apply such examinations to food being shipped across the national boundary or even within the country.

It must be realized that the purpose of acceptance sampling is to determine a course of action; acceptance decisions and analyses facilitating these decisions do not describe the quality of the remaining items in the batch. We will show later that acceptance sampling is not an appropriate means to 'control' quality in production. It will be seen that acceptance sampling applied to a series of lots (or batches) will result in there being a specified risk of accepting lots of a given quality – in other words acceptance sampling provides *quality assurance*. Nevertheless, application of acceptance sampling can lead to an improvement in quality of production. If an acceptance-sampling plan causes a supplier's production to be rejected at a high rate, the supplier may take steps to improve production methods and therefore improve quality, or otherwise the customer may be led to seek other, better sources of supply. However, although good quality of production is encouraged by a high acceptance rate, and poor quality of production is discouraged by a high rejection rate, we will show that in using such an acceptance plan there is still a possibility that a customer may receive batches of inferior quality which have been accepted by the plan.

14.1 The taking of samples

14.1.1 Random sampling

In most sampling plans, including those discussed in this book, statistical calculations are based on a number of assumptions of which two of particular significance to the food scientist are that (a) the sample of n items is randomly selected from all the items available, and (b) the microorganisms are randomly distributed throughout the product.

In order to take random samples it is necessary to use some aid for their selection. Many pocket calculators can generate random numbers, tables of random numbers are included in many books of mathematical and statistical tables (and even decahedral dice numbered 0–9 on the faces are available!).

Numbers are drawn in a form appropriate to the sampling problem under consideration. For example if the items are palletized and stacked in a warehouse, it will be necessary to use the random numbers to determine along the three spatial axes the position of each item required. In the case of product passing the inspector, for example on a conveyor belt of a production line, the random numbers will be used to indicate which item to draw after the previous item taken.

The operational difficulties of taking truly random samples from batches of food already stacked in warehouse or cold store must not be overlooked. We leave to the reader's imagination the response of a cold-store man who is asked to move pallets and boxes in order that you may select one packet randomly from the rows of pallets of boxes of packets representing a batch of many tens of thousands of packets, when he realizes that you intend to take a sample of 25 packets, with each packet likely to involve him in the extensive use of his fork-lift truck!

14.1.2 'Non-random' sampling and stratified random sampling

In certain situations it will be known that the product is heterogeneous and may be so in respect of the characteristic (e.g. a specific microorganism) being examined. Knowledge of the distribution and occurrence of the microorganism in the different areas or strata may be desired. In such cases it may be more desirable deliberately to draw samples which are not randomly chosen from the product as a whole; instead, random samples are taken from each of a number of identifiable strata. For example, this approach would be preferred if the product is kept in a refrigerated store in which considerable temperature gradients occur. The results obtained from the different strata should be separately assessed, and in the example given these results could then be checked against the data for the temperature gradients measured by use of a multichannel thermograph. If the results then indicate that the expected modification of the distribution of the quality criterion has *not* occurred, then the data could be pooled to assess overall lot quality.

14.2 Sampling plans for batches

A single-sample sampling plan needs to specify the sample size of n units to be taken, and the number of defective units c that cannot be exceeded without the lot being rejected.

When a random sample *n* is drawn without replacement from a finite lot, of size *N*, containing a specified number of defectives *m*, the calculation of the probabilities of acceptance, P_a, is made by the use of the formula for the *hypergeometric distribution*, tables of which have been published, or calculations for which can be performed using a personal computer. When P_a is plotted against p' (the fraction of defectives in a batch) the result is known as the *Operating Characteristic* (OC). The type of plot obtained by the formula for the hypergeometric distribution is discontinuous, because only integer values can be plotted on the abscissa (the *x*-axis); it is known as a *Type A* OC, *and depends on lot, or batch, size*. As the batch size increases, the number of points along the abscissa increases. In most food manufacturing operations the batch size is very large – typically many thousands – so that we can draw a continuous curve.

Some food specialities are produced in very small batch sizes, and in these cases the discontinuous nature of the distribution must be noted. A simple example of such a situation in the food industry involving a very small batch size can be considered here. One of the authors was involved in the occasional monitoring of the hygienic practices of an ice-cream chef who, in one day's work, produced up to 16 high-quality, expensive, decorative ice-cream gateaux to be supplied to three top-ranking London hotels. Making the product involved a great deal of manipulative skill so that there was a real chance of contaminants from the chef's hands being introduced into the product. Whilst on-the-spot monitoring of the hygienic technique was carried out from time to time, at other times each batch of gateaux (a day's production) would be examined by taking two of the gateaux and performing a count of *Escherichia coli* on each. A count of more than 15 *E. coli* per gram was considered unacceptable, so a gateau containing more than that concentration would be considered defective. If this count exceeded 15 per gram in both of the two units examined, then the batch would be considered unacceptable.

We can ask the question: 'What is the probability of this sampling plan accepting batches that contain four (or any other number) gateaux exceeding this count of *E. coli*?' Imagine removing the first gateau from a batch of 16 containing four defective units. Since the gateau will be cut into, even subsampling from the gateau will render it unusable by the hotels; that is, microbiological examination is destructive, and we are therefore 'sampling without replacement'. The probability of the first gateau being defective is 4 in 16; the probability of the second

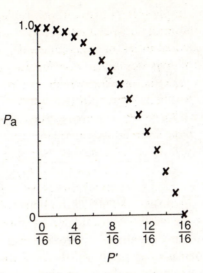

Figure 14.1 The Type A Operating Characteristic for the 2-class attributes plan $N = 16$, $n = 2$, $c = 1$.

gateau examined, after the first to be chosen was defective would therefore be 5 in 15. The probability of both gateaux being defective is thus 4/16 times 3/15 = 1/20. The Operating Characteristic of this plan is shown in Fig. 14.1.

14.3 Sampling plans for continuously running processes

A continuously running process can be considered as producing an infinite universe from which samples are drawn. Operating Characteristic curves for infinite lots are known as *Type B* OC curves (see Fig. 14.2). The process is assumed to be turning out a continuous stream of product with an average proportion of defectives p'. In this case, lots are assumed to be drawn from the continuous stream of product, and the probability of accepting a lot, P_a, will be the proportion of lots from the given process that will in the long run be accepted under the plan in which a random sample of size n will contain c or fewer defective items. This probability is given by the *binomial distribution*.

If either $p' < 0.10$, or $p'n < 5$, the *Poisson distribution* may be used as an approximation to the binomial distribution. If $p' \simeq 0.5$, the *normal*

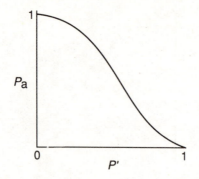

Figure 14.2 A Type B Operating Characteristic curve.

distribution provides an excellent approximation to the binomial distribution even when n is as small as 10. As the value for p' moves away from 0.5 the approximation becomes worse, but with large values of n, the normal distribution will still provide a reasonable approximation when $p'n \geq 5$, even when p' is as small as 0.10 or as large as 0.90.

14.4 Type A OC curves in food microbiology

There is only one Type B OC curve for a sampling plan of given n and c. However, there is a family of Type A Operating Characteristics, given n and c, for different values of batch size N.

As N becomes greater, the discontinuous Type A curve becomes similar in its values to the Type B curve. The Type A OC curve for $N = \infty$ is numerically identical to the Type B OC curve. When $N >$ $10n$, the Type B OC curve can be used to generate good approximations to the 'Type A' values (although the abscissa is correctly defined for a Type A curve as 'lot quality' and for a Type B curve as 'product quality'). In microbiological examinations, the destructive nature of the testing almost certainly means that $n < N/10$. Thus usually, the single Type B OC curve can be used to examine the effectiveness of the sampling plan. As already mentioned in Section 14.2, the Type A OC curve *is* applicable where the sample is drawn from a small batch size.

The perfectly discriminating sampling plan would have an OC curve as shown in Fig. 14.3. However, this curve is obtained only with 100 % inspection. In all other circumstances, where $n < N$, a lot with lot quality p'_1 may be accepted or rejected. In such cases the probability

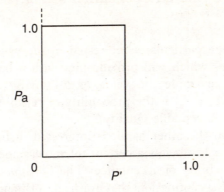

Figure 14.3 A perfectly discriminating plan, with 100 % inspection.

of acceptance P_a will be less than 1.0, but will not be reduced to zero. The OC curve thus looks like Fig. 14.4.

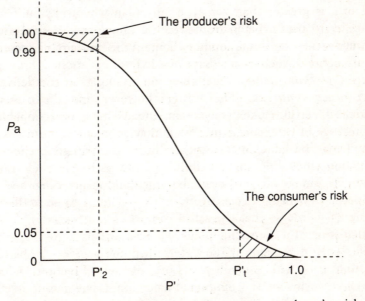

Figure 14.4 The Operating Characteristic curve, producer's risk and consumer's risk.

14.5 Producer's risk and consumer's risk (see Fig. 14.4)

A producer will be particularly interested in the value for lot quality or product quality which will provide him with a high probability of acceptance – for example the value of p'_2 giving $P_a = 0.99$. The *Producer's Risk* $(1 - P_a)$ is the probability of rejecting lots or batches that are really of Acceptable Quality.

A consumer, on the other hand, is interested in being assured that a lot with a lot quality below a certain tolerable value, p'_t, will have a suitably low probability of acceptance. The *Consumer's Risk* refers to the probability of accepting lots that are really of unacceptable quality.

14.6 Sampling plans where c = 0

For sampling plans used in conjunction with microbiological examinations for the presence of organisms considered to be highly undesirable (for example, *Salmonella* in cooked foods), a number of international organizations including ICMSF and FAO believe that it would be aesthetically and politically unacceptable to use any plan in which the value of c is greater than zero (i.e. any plan which has built in to it the ability to pass a batch from which a sample has been drawn and examined, and some units found to contain the undesirable organisms). In this context such plans have tended to be applied only to the detection of *Salmonella*, rather than, for example, to the detection of *Staphylococcus aureus*. The authors however find the presence of *S. aureus* in cream cakes and cream gateaux more objectionable than the presence of *Salmonella* in raw poultry products. Cream cakes and gateaux may be handled unhygienically by the pâtisserie chef during production (including the possibility of the pâtisserie chef using the traditional but totally unacceptable method of avoiding sputter of whipped cream being decoratively piped – namely to suck the end of the piping nozzle so that the saliva can act as a lubricant!).

Calculations for sampling plans where c equals zero are relatively simple: only n remains to be determined for a given probability of accepting a lot with a given p'_t (Lot Tolerance Fraction Defective). The three forms of the simplified equation (Harrigan & McCance, 1976) are shown below. In these plans it is conceptually easier to think about the probability of rejecting a batch with a given proportion of defectives by detecting any defective unit in the sample, so 'P_{rej}' is used here instead of 'P_a', but of course $P_a + P_{rej} = 1$.

$$P_{rej} = 1 - (1 - p')^n$$

$$p' = (1 - \sqrt[n]{(1 - P_{rej})})$$

$$n = \frac{\log(1 - P_{rej})}{\log(1 - p')}$$

These equations can, for example, be used (a) to determine the implications of particular plans for examining sterile foods for the presence of viable organisms, and (b) to calculate n for a sampling plan designed to detect a certain (low) concentration of *Salmonella* in a food.

14.6.1 The ineffectiveness of end-product examination of appertized products

In the first application mentioned above, one of the authors in his early days of employment in the food industry was asked to examine batches of incoming canned food material (that had received a botulinum cook and therefore had a high probability of being sterile!) by looking for the presence of aerobic and anaerobic bacteria in six cans from each batch. The batch would be accepted if none of the six cans was found to contain bacteria. If we ask the question as to what the proportion of defectives in the entire batch would need to be for there to be a 95 % probability of one of the six cans being defective then we get the answer:

$$p' = (1 - \sqrt[6]{(1 - 0.95)})$$

$$= 0.393$$

In other words, there would have to have been a gross failure of the heat treatment! Note that there is still a 5 % probability of accepting a batch containing nearly 40 % of defective cans!

This misconception persists. Recently the same author was involved in some overseas consultancy work, during which a very impressive dairy products factory was visited. One of the production lines was for aseptically packaged UHT-sterilized flavoured milk drinks. The laboratory staff checked the production by taking two packets from each batch of 2700 packets. These were examined for the presence of microorganisms. In this case the batch size is fairly small, but since

$N \geqslant 10n$, the Type B OC curve still provides a good approximation. Thus

$$p' = (1 - {}^{n}\sqrt{(1 - P_{\text{rej}})})$$

$$= (1 - {}^{2}\sqrt{(1 - 0.95)})$$

$$= 0.776$$

That is, this quality check will detect a gross failure of the UHT process, and not much else – for example it would be extremely unlikely to detect low concentrations of survivors of the heat-treatment, or the possibility of post-heating contamination as the result of the packaging not occurring in an aseptic environment. The quality-assurance staff had not thought of using thermograph records (thermograph chart paper was not being fitted to the thermograph), which would be a much more effective check on the efficiency of the process.

14.6.2 Use of a sampling plan to detect low concentrations of organism in a food

Suppose that we wish to apply a specification to a food such that, with a 95 % probability, batches of the foodstuff will contain fewer than one *Salmonella* per 500 g. How many 25 g units must be examined for the presence of *Salmonella*, in order to detect a level of contamination of one organism per 500 g by one of the units being found to contain *Salmonella*?

There are 20 units of 25 g in 500 g. Thus the specification we wish to apply is equivalent to there being fewer than 5 % defective 25 g units (i.e. less than 1 unit in any 20 units being positive in the batch as a whole), with a 95 % probability. The number of units, n, which needs to be taken as a sample is given by

$$n = \frac{\log(1 - 0.95)}{\log(1 - \frac{5}{100})}$$

$$= \frac{\log 0.05}{\log 0.95} = \frac{\bar{2}.6990}{\bar{1}.9777} = \frac{-1.3010}{-0.0223} = 58.3$$

That is, we need to sample 59 units, each of 25 g, all of which must be negative, in order to ensure that, in the long run, food batches contain (with a 95 % probability) fewer than one *Salmonella* per 500 g.

This is the basis for the ICMSF recommendation for dried milk and infant feeds intended for famine relief being examined by a 2-class sampling plan within which sixty 25 g units are found to be free of *Salmonella*.

14.7 Three-class attributes sampling plans

The ICMSF (1974) recommended the application of 3-class attributes sampling plans. In the particular form of the plans used by ICMSF, three parameters are specified:

n the number of units to be sampled

c_1 the number of units permitted to have counts in excess of m

$c_2 = 0$ no unit is permitted to have a count in excess of M

The values of m and M are microbiological counts such that counts of m or less can be achieved by the application of Good Manufacturing Practice and counts in excess of M represent an unacceptable microbial population on account of either a real public-health hazard, or an organoleptically detectable spoilage.

Units with counts less than m are considered to be of good quality, those with counts between m and M are considered to be of 'marginal' quality, and those with counts in excess of M are considered to be of 'bad' quality.

ICMSF (1986) have recommended microbiological specifications for foods based upon the use of 3-class and 2-class plans, with the details of the plan being determined by the nature of the hazard (see Table 14.1). An example of such a specification is given in Table 14.2. Specifications of the same form are being recommended by the Codex Alimentarius Committees of the FAO.

14.8 Sampling plans based on variables

The principal advantages of the 2-class and 3-class attributes sampling plans described above are that they are simple to apply, and that although the 3-class plans make fuller use than the 2-class plans of the microbial counts, they are still reasonably robust in that they do not make any assumption about the nature of the distribution of the

Table 14.1 Suggested sampling plans for combinations of degrees of health and conditions of use (i.e. the 15 'cases'). From ICMSF, 1986

Degree of concern relative to utility and health hazard	Conditions in which food is expected to be handled and consumed after sampling, in the usual course of events		
	Conditions reduce degree of concern	Conditions cause no change in concern	Conditions may increase concern
No direct health hazard Utility, e.g. shelf-life and spoilage	Increase shelf-life Case 1 3-class $n=5$, $c=3$	No change Case 2 3-class $n=5$, $c=2$	Reduce shelf-life Case 3 3-class $n=5$, $c=1$
Health hazard Low, indirect (indicator)	Reduce hazard Case 4 3-class $n=5$, $c=3$	No change Case 5 3-class $n=5$, $c=2$	Increase hazard Case 6 3-class $n=5$, $c=1$
Moderate, direct, limited spread	Case 7 3-class $n=5$, $c=2$	Case 8 3-class $n=5$, $c=1$	Case 9 3-class $n=10$, $c=1$
Moderate, direct, potentially extensive spread	Case 10 2-class $n=5$, $c=0$	Case 11 2-class $n=10$, $c=0$	Case 12 2-class $n=20$, $c=0$
Severe, direct	Case 13 2-class $n=15$, $c=0$	Case 14 2-class $n=30$, $c=0$	Case 15 2-class, $n=60$, $c=0$

Table 14.2 Recommended microbiological specifications for pasteurized liquid, frozen and dried egg products (ICMSF, 1986)

Test	Case	Plan class	n	c	Limit per gram m	M
Aerobic mesophilic count	2	3	5	2	5×10^4	10^6
Coliforms	5	3	5	2	10^1	10^3
Salmonella	10	2	5	0	0	–
normal routine	11	2	10	0	0	–
	12	2	20	0	0	–
Salmonella	10	2	15	0	0	–
for high-risk	11	2	30	0	0	–
populations	12	2	60	0	0	–

Notes: The case number for *Salmonella* is chosen according to whether the expected use of the product will reduce, cause no change in, or increase concern (see Table 14.1). For foods intended for high-risk populations, the case number remains the same, but n is increased to increase stringency.

microorganisms in the batch of food. In order to make full use of the data being obtained in microbiological examinations it would be necessary to set specifications based on variables plans. Unfortunately, to apply variables plans correctly it is necessary to know how the microorganisms are distributed in the food; most variables plans are based on the assumption that the microorganisms will be log-normally distributed (i.e. the logarithms of the counts will conform to a normal distribution). Variables plans will be invalid if the assumption made about the distribution of the microorganisms is incorrect. Thus, if using a variables plan, it is necessary to test the observed variance against the assumed variance. Smelt & Quadt (1990) suggested a procedure for the design of variables plans which requires only two replicates from each batch to be examined ($n = 2$) to give an almost identical operating characteristic to a 3-class attributes plan with five replicates ($n = 5$). This is achieved by comparing current data with previous sets of data. A χ^2 test is used to compare the observed variances with the variance previously determined on at least five replicates from at least 10 different batches; as long as there is not a significant deviation from the assumed distribution then the variables plan can be validly applied to the batch under test.

At present, variables plans have not been widely adopted for recommended or legal microbiological specifications for foods.

— 15

The use of control charts and confidence limits

In Chapter 9, we suggested that there are three broad types of laboratory, each with a probable different requirement for data analysis. We have discussed the first of these in Chapter 14, and now we want to look at the application of control charts and of confidence limits.

15.1 Control charts

In any production process some variation in quality is unavoidable. The variation can be divided into two categories:

(1) random variation;

(2) variation due to assignable causes – that is, causes over which we have some degree of control (e.g. fluctuations in process temperature).

If variation due to one or more assignable causes is present in the output from a process, the process is said to be *out of control*. The control chart enables us to define the state of statistical control, and enables us to judge when it has been attained or when it has been lost.

A sample of n units is taken at frequent intervals and a chart kept of, for example, sample mean against time. There are different types of control chart depending on whether we are measuring a continuous variable, the 'fraction defective', number of defects per unit, etc. but they are all quite similar.

If one variable is measured it can be assumed to have a normal distribution when the process is under statistical control. The presence of assignable causes of variation would then show up in the data as variation outside the usual range for a normally distributed variable. This can usually be attributed to a change in either the population mean (μ) or the standard deviation (σ) of the normal distribution for the measured variable. To detect a change in μ we could construct a control chart of the sample mean ($\bar{x}$) against time; to detect a change in σ we could plot the sample variance (s^2) against time, although it is easier to plot the range R against time.

15.1.1 Statistical procedure for setting up $\bar{x}$:t control charts

The statistical 'procedure' is as follows:

1. From past data obtain good estimates of μ and σ.

2. Estimate the standard error of $\bar{x}$ as σ/n.

3. From tables of the normal distribution it can be determined that if a process be in control, then only one point in a thousand should be above the value ($\mu + 3.09\sigma/n$).

   This would be assigned as the *Upper Action Limit* for the $\bar{x}$ chart. For a variable which it is desired to be close to a preferred value, for example weight or size, one would also specify a lower action limit.

   In the case of undesirable microorganisms only upper limits are specified, but the lower limit may be useful to indicate, through results falling below it, a possible failure in techniques or media for growing the organism (although such results could of course also indicate that the process was in fact turning out product of better microbiological quality).

4. If a point falls above the Upper Action Limit, it is probable that assignable causes of variation are present (e.g. a sudden failure in the effectiveness of a pasteurization process), and action to trace and eliminate these causes should be initiated.

5. In order to improve the sensitivity of the control charts an *Upper Warning Limit* can be drawn in at the value ($\mu + 1.96\sigma/n$).

6. When the process is in control, one point in 40 can be expected to be above the Upper Warning Limit. Two successive points, or more than 1 in 40, above this limit can be taken as good evidence

that assignable causes of variation are present in the process.

When setting up a control chart, good estimates of μ and σ are required, so at least 25 groups of observations should be obtained. The mean, $\bar{x}$, of each group is calculated, and the averages of means then calculated. The average of the means is taken as an estimate of μ.

The action and warning limits should then be drawn as described above, and the groups of data that have already been used to estimate μ and σ should be inspected in relation to these limits. If any of the groups lie outside the limits as described above, then these groups should be deleted, and μ, σ, and the two limits re-estimated from those remaining. The groups remaining should now fall within the newly estimated limits. If any groups fall outside the newly estimated limits, or if a large proportion of the original complete set of groups fell outside the original limits, then the process is out of control and the limits cannot yet be calculated.

15.1.2 Use of the $\bar{x}$:t control chart

Once a chart has been set up with the Upper Action Limit, Upper Warning Limit, and μ marked on it, new results should be entered on it as they are gathered and determined (see Fig. 15.1a). In addition, any important known changes in the process should also be marked on the charts; for example a new operator, a new supplier of raw material used in the food production (even a new supplier of microbiological medium used in the tests) (see Fig. 15.1b).

Lack of control can be indicated by:

(1) occasional points falling above the Upper Action Limit;

(2) too many points falling above the Upper Warning Limit;

(3) a *gradual* change to a new value of μ or σ, or both (see Fig. 15.1c) as might be seen if ineffective cleaning permitted a build-up of microorganisms on the equipment;

(4) a *sudden* unexpected change to a new value of μ or σ, or both, which can occur through change to a new supplier, for example.

One aspect that needs to be considered in the context of microbiological analyses is that the food microbiologist may wish to define a Warning Limit or an Action Limit in relation to the public health implications of the counts, whatever the position in relation to the statistical values.

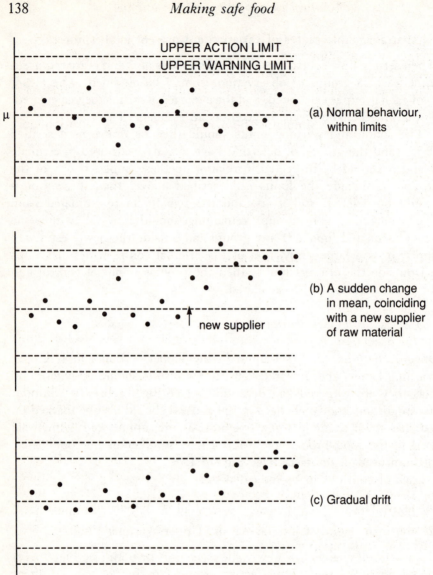

Figure 15.1 The $\bar{x}:t$ control chart.

If $(\mu + 3.09\sigma/n)$ is greater than the number of microorganisms acknowledged to be of public-health concern, then this will require reconsideration of either the production process, or the method of analysis (which could also be contributing to the amount of variation in the data), or both, before control chart procedures can be used to provide early warning of poor quality.

Operating characteristic (OC) curves and Average Run Length (ARL, i.e. the average number of batches or items sampled until one is 'rejected') can be calculated for these control charts.

This brief introduction to the design of simple control charts considers the $\bar{x}:t$ chart only. One other type of control chart which may be used to advantage is the Cumulative Sum (CUSUM) Chart. This is more sensitive than the $\bar{x}$-chart to slight changes in the mean. Further information on $\bar{x}$-charts, CUSUM and other types of control charts can be found in Wetherill (1977), Ryan (1989), and Oakland & Followell (1990), and additional information on decision-making with CUSUM charts is provided by Lucas (1973, 1976, 1982).

15.2 Calculation of confidence intervals on viable counts

15.2.1 Colony counts

The microbiologist is always advised not to place too much reliance on a colony count of a mixed microbial population if the number of colonies on a standard 8–9 cm diameter Petri dish exceeds around 300, since with colonial concentrations exceeding this figure the count will usually be depressed to an unknown degree by overcrowding and microbial antagonism. However, provided that these microbiological errors do not occur, the statistical error is reduced the more colonies that are counted. When replicate plates have been prepared at each dilution, the arithmetic mean at the chosen dilution (the *lowest* dilution that results in fewer than 300 colonies per standard Petri dish) is used to calculate the microbial concentration in the original sample. The *statistical* reliability of the count can be assessed by determining the 95 % confidence interval (c.i.). This range is given by

$$\frac{(n\bar{x} \pm 1.96\sqrt{(n\bar{x})}}{n}$$

where n is the number of plates at the dilution chosen

$\bar{x}$ is the arithmetic mean of the colony count at that dilution

[and $(n\bar{x})$ is therefore the total number of colonies counted on all the plates at the chosen dilution].

The fewer the colonies counted, the wider will be the 95 % confidence interval. Usually the reliability of the count becomes unacceptable if

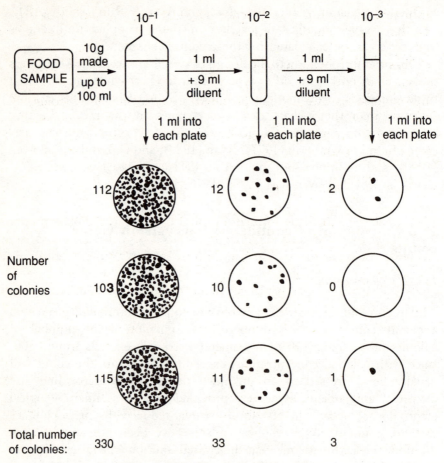

Figure 15.2 The pour plate count.

fewer than around 30 colonies are counted. Maximum practical precision is obtained in crucial situations by counting around 600 colonies (which may require between 2 and 15 replicate plates at the chosen dilution), but often in routine microbiological analyses of foods the counting of around 100 colonies will give a perfectly acceptable level of confidence.

Some fundamental, though simple, principles of the colony-counting procedure deserve great emphasis because they are not sufficiently appreciated. Let us suppose that we had prepared a plate count on a food sample, with the results shown in Fig. 15.2. To estimate the count we can use the 10^{-1} dilution, the average count being 110 colony-forming units (c.f.u. – see Section 12.3), giving an estimate of 1.1×10^3 c.f.u. g^{-1}. The 95 % c.i. is

$$\frac{330 \pm 1.96\sqrt{330}}{3} \simeq 980\text{--}1220 \text{ c.f.u. } g^{-1}.$$

But suppose that we had not prepared plates at the 10^{-1} dilution, and that the estimated count of 1.1×10^3 c.f.u. g^{-1} had been obtained by counting 33 colonies on three plates at the 10^{-2} dilution. The 95 % c.i. would then be

$$\frac{33 \pm 1.96\sqrt{33}}{3} \simeq 730\text{--}1470 \text{ c.f.u. } g^{-1}.$$

A similar calculation performed on the 3 colonies at the 10^{-3} dilution will show that decisions should not be taken on counts derived from so few colonies, as the 95 % c.i. in this case is from '0' to 2130 c.f.u. g^{-1}. It is also not microbiologically sensible to rely on a count derived from only one or two colonies per plate. In most quality-assurance laboratories most plate counts are not prepared in the sterile atmosphere of a laminar flow or Class II cabinet, but at the open bench. As long as a couple of hundred colonies are counted on a plate, a possible slight airborne contamination leading to one additional colony on the plate will distort the count by less than 1 %. The same amount of contamination of one additional c.f.u. on to a plate which receives only one c.f.u. from the sample dilution will double the perceived microbiological content of the food sample.

Preparing replicate plates on more than one dilution is likely to permit the choice of a dilution which leads to an acceptably narrow 95 % c.i. In addition, it is also likely to provide an opportunity for detecting some types of operator error or experimental error. For example, if instead of the 330 colonies at the 10^{-1} dilution there had been no colonies, although there were 33 colonies at the 10^{-2} dilution, one possible explanation which could be further investigated is that the food contains a microbistatic compound which was diluted to below the minimum inhibitory concentration before the microorganisms were diluted out to below the level detected by the procedure. Conversely, obtaining 330 colonies at the 10^{-1} dilution, but no colonies at subsequent dilutions, could be due to the worker forgetting to transfer the inoculum along the dilution series, or to the food containing a nutrient which supplements a medium that is nutritionally deficient for the microorganisms present in the food.

Table 15.1 Values of the MPN for three tubes inoculated from each of three successive decimal dilutions (Harrigan & McCance, 1976)

Number of positive tubes observed at each dilution			MPN* of microorganisms per inoculum of the first dilution	Category†
1st dilution	2nd dilution	3rd dilution		
0	0	0	0	–
0	0	1	0.3	3
0	1	0	0.3	2
0	1	1	0.6	4
0	2	0	0.6	4
1	0	0	0.4	1
1	0	1	0.7	3
1	0	2	1.1	4
1	1	0	0.7	2
1	1	1	1.1	4
1	2	0	1.1	3
1	2	1	1.5	4
1	3	0	1.6	4
2	0	0	0.9	1
2	0	1	1.4	3
2	0	2	2.0	4
2	1	0	1.5	2
2	1	1	2.0	4
2	1	2	3.0	4
2	2	0	2.0	3
2	2	1	3.0	4
2	2	2	3.5	4
2	2	3	4.0	4
2	3	0	3.0	4
2	3	1	3.5	4
2	3	2	4.0	4
3	0	0	2.5	1
3	0	1	4.0	2
3	0	2	6.5	4
3	1	0	4.5	1

Table 15. 1 – Continued

Number of positive tubes observed at each dilution			MPN* of microorganisms per inoculum of the first dilution	Category†
1st dilution	2nd dilution	3rd dilution		
3	1	1	7.5	2
3	1	2	11.5	3
3	1	3	16.0	4
3	2	0	9.5	1
3	2	1	15.0	2
3	2	2	20.0	3
3	2	3	30.0	4
3	3	0	25.0	1
3	3	1	45.0	1
3	3	2	110.0	1
3	3	3	>140.0	–

*Approximate 95 % confidence limits may be calculated as suggested by Cochran (1950) as MPN/4.68 to MPN × 4.68.

†In the long run, Category 1 combinations may be expected to constitute 67.5 % of test results containing both positive and negative tubes; categories (1 + 2) 91 %; and categories (1 + 2 + 3) 99 % of such test results. Category 4 and unlisted combinations are highly unlikely (Woodward, 1957). Combinations from categories 3 and 4 should not be used as the basis for quality assurance decisions involving the rejection and/or reprocessing of batches of food – samples should be retested. In the event of large numbers of improbable combinations being obtained, experimental procedures should be examined closely, as this is indicative of the presence of disturbing influences and poor experimental procedures – for example improper mixing of samples and/or dilutions, presence of antagonistic substances in the foodstuffs, etc.

It should be noted that it is not statistically legitimate or meaningful to calculate the mean counts from more than one dilution and then to average these means. There *are* statistical procedures for using the data from more than one dilution, by calculating *weighted means*, but the effort involved in determining the weighting to be given will usually outweigh the benefit obtained.

If using a procedure (e.g. Miles & Misra surface drop counts) which results in the incubation of an inoculated drop of agar of small diameter, the maximum number of colonies from a mixed population that will be microbiologically acceptable will often be between 10 and 30. In such cases one must not be deterred from obtaining counts of sufficient

Table 15.2 Factors for calculating approximate 95 % confidence intervals on MPNs derived from multiple tube counts (Cochran, 1950)

Number of tubes at each dilution	Dilution ratio			
	2	4	5	10
1	4.00	7.14	8.32	14.45
2	2.67	4.00	4.47	6.61
3	2.23	3.10	3.39	4.68
4	2.00	2.68	2.88	3.80
5	1.86	2.41	2.58	3.30
6	1.76	2.23	2.38	2.98
7	1.69	2.10	2.23	2.74
8	1.64	2.00	2.12	2.57
9	1.58	1.92	2.02	2.43
10	1.55	1.86	1.95	2.32

colonies because of the constraints of the method; more replicates must be made to achieve an appropriate level of confidence in the result.

15.2.2 Most Probable Number (MPN) counts

The MPN count provides, by a statistical technique, an estimate of the viable population in a sample, usually by using growth, or some quality such as acid production, in tubes of liquid medium (also known as a multiple tube count). Tubes containing the liquid medium are inoculated with, for example, 1-ml quantities of serial dilutions of the material being investigated. After incubation, the highest dilution giving growth (or the appropriate reaction, such as acid and gas production) is noted, and this enables an estimate of bacterial numbers in the original sample to be made. For example, if growth occurs in a tube inoculated with 1 ml of a 10^{-2} dilution, but not in a tube inoculated with 1 ml of a 10^{-3} dilution there were probably at least 100 but not as many as 1000 bacteria per millilitre or per gram of the original sample. In practice, several tubes are inoculated at each dilution, and the set of three consecutive (usually decimal) dilutions chosen which includes the dilution at which around half of the tubes show growth or reaction and around half do not, together with the dilution on each side of this 'target' dilution. The MPN to result in this combination of positive and negative tubes is obtained by reference to statistical tables. Commonly in food microbiology, a decimal dilution series is prepared, and three or five tubes inoculated at each dilution (see Table 15.1).

It should be noted that Table 15.1 indicates the most probable number of organisms in the inoculum of the first dilution of the set of three chosen for the estimation, *given the correctness of certain assumptions about the randomness of the distribution of the organisms in the samples and in the dilutions thereof*. Many MPN tables do not indicate whether such a combination of positive and negative tubes is *itself* probable. Woodward (1957) listed the likelihoods of the various combinations, in the form of four categories of result, and these were incorporated into the MPN tables given by Harrigan & McCance (1976) (see Table 15.1). As can be seen from the footnote to Table 15.1, the categorization shown in these MPN tables enables laboratory workers to monitor their laboratory technique.

In addition, a 95 % confidence interval can be calculated for an MPN. Cochran (1950) provided a simple technique for obtaining a rough estimate of the 95 % confidence interval (see Tables 15.1 and 15.2). In fact, the confidence interval will depend in a rather complex manner on the numbers and positions of the positive tubes. Accurate confidence intervals can be calculated with a computer or programmable calculator and de Man (1975, 1977) has listed 95 and 99 % confidence intervals for results from single MPN tests and for results forming one of a series of MPN tests. de Man's (1975) 3-tube table was reproduced by ICMSF (1978). Tillett (1987) pointed out that these confidence intervals are based on the same assumptions made in the calculation of MPN tables and that if the nature of the distribution of the microorganisms in the material being examined is not known, it is more appropriate to calculate a 'Most Probable Range' rather than an MPN. However, national or international specifications or standards would need to be framed in such a way as to permit the use of MPR as well as MPN estimations.

All the aforementioned considerations of the confidence that one has in the count derive from probability theory, but there are also biological sources of error. For example, the number of microorganisms in a sample will be much underestimated if more than one microorganism is required to initiate growth in a tube.

16

The Hazard Analysis Critical Control Point system and its implementation

16.1 Introduction

In Chapter 14 we considered the application of microbiological specifications to food materials and end-products and the related investigations. A different approach to determining and improving microbiological quality is directly to ascertain the quality of hygienic practices by inspecting factories and the production processes. Within a country, a government agency may be able to use a factory inspection system very effectively. In the UK this approach has traditionally been the one adopted by the local government Environmental Health Officers and in the USA it is the basis for the Federal Codes of GMP. Of course factory inspection may not be a feasible proposition for a government agency concerned about the quality of a food being imported into the country from another, perhaps distant, country. Nevertheless, an assurance about the hygienic quality of production of food moving in international trade can be obtained from the fact that a factory is certificated under the *ISO 9000* series; the implications and importance of certification have been discussed in Chapter 10.

The two approaches, application of specifications and the inspection of production procedures and facilities, can be considered to be complementary, and a careful distribution of available funds between them is likely to provide the consumer with the best protection. The distribution of funds which will give the best cost–benefit ratio will depend on the nature of the food product, the most important hazards, the movement of the food in national and international markets, and many socio-economic aspects.

In an attempt to formalize the procedures for in-factory inspection in the USA, the Federal Food and Drugs Administration (USFDA) attempted to define and delineate their inspection system by adopting the Hazard Analysis Critical Control Point (HACCP) concept which was developed by the National Aeronautics and Space Administration, the US Army Natick Laboratories, and the Pillsbury Company. Of course, many food companies have for a very long time monitored Good Manufacturing Practice (GMP), which includes hygienic practices and cleaning and disinfection regimes, by in-factory monitoring, inspections and checks. Microbiological analysis of the end-product by an examination of representative samples from the batch can then be used to confirm (or otherwise!) the effectiveness of the GMP procedures and of their monitoring.

Many food companies have realized the advantages of conducting in-factory inspections by using a standardized and formalized system similar to the HACCP procedures adopted by the USFDA, and the ICMSF devoted *Microorganisms in Foods, Volume 4* to a discussion of HACCP. Those seeking certification under the *ISO 9000* series frequently use HACCP or a very similar system for examining their hygienic standards. Mayes & Kilsby (1989) have advocated the use of HAZOP (Hazard and Operability Studies) analysis, and Mossel & van Netten (1990) discussed the use of LISA (Longitudinally Integrated Safety Assurance).

16.2 Principles of the HACCP system

As the name suggests, the system involves the following essential stages:

1. Hazard Analysis, which consists in identifying and evaluating the hazards arising from ingredients, key processes, distribution and retailing, and various relevant human factors including the probable use of the food product.

2. A determination of the Critical Control Points (CCPs), which are defined as the points in the production process at which the identified Hazards can be effectively controlled. An alternative definition of Critical Control Points emphasizes the need for the

continuous integrity of the CCPs: this definition is that CCPs are processing determinants whose loss of control permits the realization of the potential hazard as an unacceptable food safety or food spoilage risk.

3. Establishment of appropriate systems to monitor these CCPs.

In the implementation of the system, however, there is likely to be an additional initial stage in which a flow-chart of the manufacturing process for a product is drawn up, on which the Hazards and CCPs can then be indicated. The four phases are thus:

1. Construction of a flow-chart of the entire process (this may include the distribution, warehousing and retail operations if appropriate).

2. Identification of Hazards, and the location of these recorded at the appropriate point on the flow-chart.

3. Identification of Critical Control Points, and location of these on the flow-chart, followed by a re-evaluation of the interaction between Hazards and CCPs.

4. Listing and evaluation of the monitoring and QA Procedures used to ensure continuing efficacy of control at the CCPs, together with a consideration of the nature of the documentation on monitoring and QA procedures and the storage of this documentation.

Inspectors from governmental and other external agencies carrying out HACCP inspections will usually get rapidly familiar with the various aspects to be identified and evaluated, so they may use a proforma check-list which combines all these phases under headings that relate to the different areas of the factory and of production. They will thus not need to undertake four separate tours of inspection of the factory. This short-cut may be necessary from the point of view of funding or staffing levels in the agency which will usually have a large number of manufacturing premises to oversee. However, for anybody relatively new to HACCP inspections we would recommend that these four different phases are considered separately, and a separate tour of inspection used to consider the elements of each phase. In the case of company QA staff, it would be preferable for even those who are familiar with HACCP evaluation to keep the different phases of the operation separate, as it is easy to overlook important details if attempting to cover too much in one tour of inspection.

16.3 The microbiological principles involved

In order to carry out an effective HACCP inspection, the inspector needs a good understanding of the factors determining the occurrence, growth, survival or death of microorganisms in foods. Mossel & Ingram (1955) provided a comprehensive listing of these factors. A summary list can be made as follows:

1. The food and the process

    (a) The innate infection of the raw materials

    (b) Contamination during handling and from equipment

    (c) The chemical and physical properties of the raw materials

        (i)   Chemical composition – nutrients and antimicrobial substances

        (ii)   Microheterogeneity of the material

        (iii) pH and buffering power

        (iv) Gaseous balance

        (v)   Oxidation–reduction potential (Eh)

        (vi) a_w

        (vii) Mechanical barriers

    (d) Transport and preprocessing storage conditions

        (i)   Temperature

        (ii)   Gaseous environment

        (iii) Humidity

        (iv) Time

    (e) Processing and preservation procedures

        (i)   Direct: temperature, added chemicals, irradiation etc.

        (ii)   Indirect: chemical and physical changes produced in the food

    (f) Packaging and post-processing storage conditions

        (i)   Temperature

    (ii)   Gaseous environment

    (iii) Humidity

    (iv) Time

2. The microorganisms concerned

    (g) Characteristics of the species/strain

        (i)   Resistance to lethal processes

        (ii)   Tolerance of inhibitory factors

        (iii) Optimum requirements for growth

        (iv) Growth rate

    (h) Synergistic effects between microorganisms

        (i)   Changes in structure and physical properties of the food

        (ii)   Supply of additional nutrients and growth factors

        (iii) Changes in pH and gaseous environment

    (i) Antagonistic effects between microorganisms

        (i)   Competition for nutrients

        (ii)   Changes in pH and gaseous environment

        (iii) Production of antibiotics, etc.

16.4 Implementation of the HACCP system

In Section 16.2 it was pointed out that a HACCP assessment essentially consisted in four phases. We will now consider each of these phases in turn.

16.4.1 Phase 1: construction of the flow-chart

A generalized flow-chart such as that shown in Fig. 16.1 can be used to indicate the type of item that needs to be looked for when constructing the detailed and specific flow-chart relating to a particular product being made in a particular factory. Figure 16.2 shows a similar generalized flow-chart, but with the typical QA functions found in most factories. An example of a product-specific flow-chart is shown in Fig. 16.3, but this would be considerably modified by the particular layout and procedures found in the specific factory being examined. This would represent only the first stage of the construction of the detailed chart. ICMSF suggest that the construction of the detailed flow-chart containing all the data required for Phase 2 requires a team of at least two specialists – a food microbiologist and a process engineer. A real flow-chart showing the meat pie production in a given factory will need to display many other things. For example, in the hypothetical example shown in Fig. 16.3, amongst the important data to obtain would be:

1. The method of transport of the raw materials, transit times and temperatures. This would be important if the supplier of the raw materials were applying 'end-product' microbiological examinations to his output (the supplier's 'end product' is the meat pie manufacturer's starting material), and the meat pie manufacturer was making use of such quality data in determining the fitness for use of the raw material.

2. The times and temperatures of storage of the various categories of raw materials.

3. The make and model of equipment being used in processing and manufacture, together with the relevant technical details of its operation. For example, the choppers and mixers used to prepare the meat mix could have an effect in the time taken to prepare the mix, the temperatures attained during mixing (some mixers are cooled, others rely on any cooling coming from ice or chilled water that is incorporated into the mix). If there is more than one make or model of a piece of equipment available for a given operation, and there is a tendency to use whichever one is free at the time, this could have an important influence on the quality of the product – for example the fineness of chopping and mixing, the ease of cleaning the equipment, and so on. One important aid to minimizing quality variations is to have specific items of equipment specified for each product line.

4. Any holding times or identifiable 'bottlenecks' in the production line. These may occur when, for example, the pie-making machine has a much faster throughput than has the travelling oven. If there is as a result a build-up of racks of uncooked pies, what then happens to them? If they are kept in the bakery department next to the travelling

152

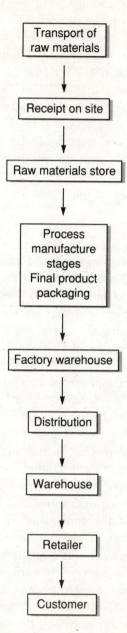

Figure 16.1 Generalized flow-chart of typical production process.

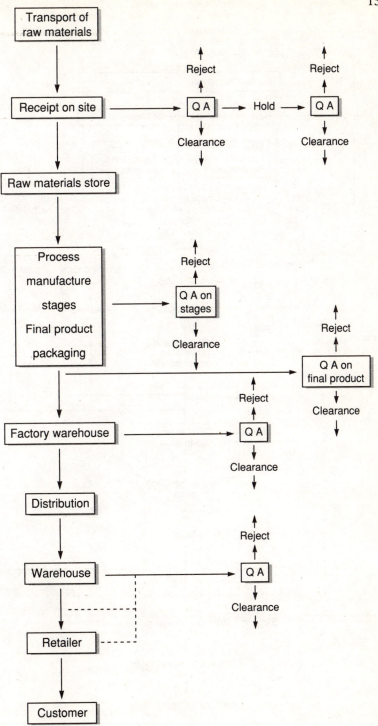

Figure 16.2 Flow-chart of typical production process.

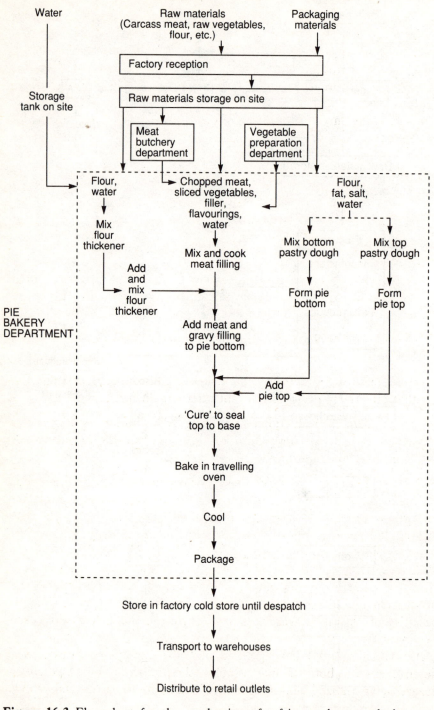

Figure 16.3 Flow-chart for the production of refrigerated pre-cooked meat pies.

oven awaiting their turn, how long may they remain there, and what is their eventual temperature before baking? If the build-up in pies continues, towards the end of the day, may they then be placed in a cold store until the next day and then baked immediately on removal from the cold store? In one well-known example, failure to achieve a 'botulinum cook' in a canning factory was due to this sort of problem: a mismatching in the capacity of the can-filling and sealing machines on the one hand and the retorts on the other. Filled cans which were consequently cold-stored until they could be processed were not sufficiently heat-treated on subsequent cooking because the lower starting temperature had not been taken into account.

16.4.2 Phase 2: Hazard Analysis

There are four general types of microbiological hazard:

1. Raw materials or food ingredients which can be regarded as potential sources of pathogens, food poisoning organisms, food spoilage organisms, or toxic substances (e.g. pre-formed toxins).

2. Sources of contamination during production, processing or distribution.

3. Manufacturing processes which lack a controlled processing step that effectively destroys relevant microorganisms.

4. Steps during production, processing, distribution, storage, etc. which provide an opportunity for microorganisms to survive or even grow and multiply.

The Hazard Analysis requires these various elements to be evaluated. It should be noted that microbial characteristics will affect the relative importance of the hazard groups listed above. For example, in the case of a foodborne pathogen that cannot multiply in the food and that has a low infective dose (e.g. *Campylobacter*, viruses), whether or not a food is refrigerated is not of great direct relevance. Thus, Hazard Analysis requires the food microbiologist to examine all aspects of the production as illustrated on the detailed flow-chart, using an evaluation based on an informed awareness of the determinants listed before (see Section 16.3).

As ICMSF (1988) have pointed out, the analysis requires also a determination of both the *risk*, which is the probability of the potential hazard being realized, and its *severity*. This is important in establishing a rank order of points requiring consideration. The difference between GMP and HACCP lies partly in the inclusion in the latter of an assessment of which aspects should have the highest priority.

Sometimes there will be a difference in the risk and severity aspects according to the country. For example, the survival of the more thermoduric thermophilic spore-formers such as *Bacillus stearothermophilus* and *Bacillus coagulans* is of much greater significance in a country with a tropical or sub-tropical climate than in a country with a temperate climate. In the latter countries, these organisms are used in the canned food industry primarily as 'indicators' of inadequate heat treatment, or as 'index organisms' relating to the possible presence of *Clostridium botulinum* because (unless the company is intending to export to a tropical country) storage temperatures are unlikely to be high enough for growth to occur. However, in tropical or sub-tropical regions the organisms are significant as spoilage organisms in their own right.

Obviously there is a cost factor involved in any control steps to be taken, and in some cases the cost of controlling a low-severity low-risk hazard may be judged to be too high. Unfortunately, in many countries the general population has not been adequately informed by their governments of the nature of cost-risk assessments, and this will often cause ill-informed social and political considerations to predominate in the decision-making process, for example in reply to unrealistic pleas for there to be no *Salmonella* in raw poultry.

16.4.3 Phase 3: Critical Control Points

A Critical Control Point may provide a total elimination of one or more microbiological hazard, and ICMSF (1988) has designated such a CCP as a *CCP1*. In other cases, a Critical Control Point may reduce a microbiological hazard without entirely eliminating it, and this has been designated by the ICMSF as a *CCP2*.

The efficacy of a CCP may be very dependent on the non-variability of the production process – a minor variation in the process or procedures away from the production and process parameters determined and identified during the construction of the flow-chart may have a disproportionately large effect on a CCP (e.g. addition of particulate sugar rather than sugar syrup to fruit for canning, which causes localized reductions in a_w and consequent increases in the heating required to destroy the microorganisms in those areas). Thus part of the quality management of the factory is to ensure that there is a standardization in the production and process parameters, and that deviation from these does not occur without identification and re-evaluation.

The choice of an appropriate CCP requires a good understanding of microbiology and of microbial ecology. For example, *Clostridium perfringens* food poisoning is often caused in institutional catering by the cooking and slow cooling of large bulks of meat or meat dishes (Chapter 4). It would be inappropriate to attempt to deal with this problem by examining the raw meat for the presence of *C. perfringens*, even when the meat concerned is frozen, and the microbiological results could be obtained whilst holding the batch in frozen storage. This is because *C. perfringens* spores can be expected as contaminants of raw meat. The appropriate measures to take to prevent such outbreaks of food poisoning relate to the prescription of the maximum amount of the meat or meat dish that can be cooked in one piece or volume, and, if the food is not to be eaten immediately, the definition of adequately rapid cooling procedures in terms of the cooling rates to be achieved. (A similar situation arises in the case of salmonella enteritis caused by spit-roasted or barbecued poultry, since it is unlikely that a source of *Salmonella*-free poultry can be assured, unless the poultry meat has been subjected to irradiation.)

Some examples of CCPs are shown in a simplified flow-chart in Fig. 16.4.

16.4.4 Phase 4: Monitoring and QC procedures, and documentation

16.4.4.1 Monitoring and QC procedures

Monitoring the CCPs and taking Control Action will be the ultimate responsibility of the QA department, but as already discussed in Chapters 9 and 10 it is advantageous to involve all staff actively in quality, so that first-level monitoring can often be undertaken by workers on the production line. In this case it is important that bonus payments are not determined by amount of output, as a critical deviation in a CCP parameter will sometimes cause loss of output, reprocessing or a temporary line stoppage. If the entire staff are to be motivated in quality management then quality criteria should be at least as important as amount of output in determining bonus payments (see Chapter 10).

Some CCPs can be continuously monitored. For example, a heat treatment can be examined by the use of thermocouples, with thermographs giving a permanent hard copy of the data, but in addition

Hazards   **Primary CCPs**

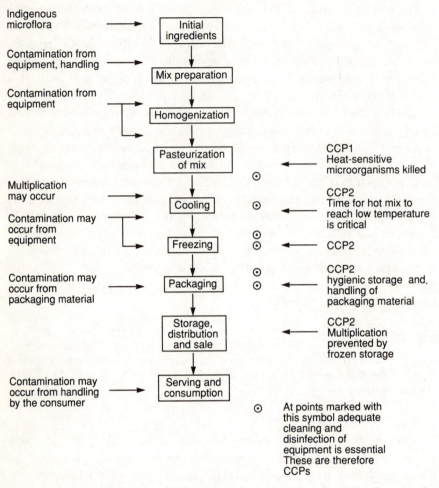

Figure 16.4 Simplified HACCP flow-chart of the production of a simple ice-cream.

there can be electronic feedback, for example the automatic continuous computation of the F-value of a continuous heating process (e.g. in a UHT sterilization plant). There can also be audible and/or visual alarms with product diversion procedures that can be quite sophisticated. These physical methods of monitoring, which are non-destructive, contrast with microbiological examinations, which are destructive

(Chapter 14). Furthermore, microbiological testing is normally of little value for monitoring CCPs during production, because of the delay before results are known. Microbiological examinations of the raw materials can, however, prove extremely useful, especially when the test-time is a small fraction of the shelf-life of the raw material; for example spore counts can be used on dried ingredients to be incorporated into canned food products.

The documented monitoring, control and action procedures should precisely state:

(1) who is responsible for each monitoring procedure;

(2) under what circumstances action is to be taken;

(3) what are the quantitative limits on the data derived from the monitoring procedure which require action to be taken;

(4) what that action is to be; and finally

(5) what are the documentary procedures to report the action.

16.4.4.2 Documentation
Documentation needs to be produced on four or even five levels:

Level 1: *The Company Quality Manual* will include the company's Quality Policy, and define the company objectives, strategy and plan for quality management. In the microbiological context it is likely to describe the way in which HACCP analyses and assessments are to be carried out, and may provide proforma check-lists for this purpose.

Level 2: *The Factory Quality Manual* will give the factory-specific and product-specific QA procedures, based on the HACCP assessments which have been carried out for each product. Specific descriptions will be given. For example in the case of the cleaning and disinfection procedures to be applied within the factory, for each item of equipment there will be a prescription of the frequency of the cleaning processes, the choice and concentration of the detergent-sanitizers to be used, and the monitoring procedures to be adopted to determine the efficacy of the cleaning process.

Level 3: *Departmental Procedures* will be limited to the specific procedures required within that section of the factory. A manual of this type will also be required for the QA department itself, not only describing the monitoring procedures that the QA department will be applying throughout the factory, but also describing the monitoring procedures to be applied *within* the laboratory (e.g. nature and frequency of checks on incubators and water-baths, checks on efficacy of media, etc.).

Level 4: *Individual Work Instruction Sheets* will give each factory operative a description and timetable of all the procedures which he or she is expected to carry out. It is important to make these accurate but succinct and in non-technical language: the operatives themselves should be closely involved in producing these instruction sheets.

Level 5: *Monitoring Documents* will include laboratory data books listing results of microbiological examinations, control charts, thermograph records, records of materials and suppliers, etc. It is important that all of these can be related to the relevant specific batch numbers of the various food products.

16.5 Towards improved products

Throughout this book we have presented the various factors to be borne in mind by those responsible, directly or indirectly, for the management of the microbiological quality of foods. HACCP provides a good framework for bringing microbiological expertise to bear on the manufacture, distribution and storage of food products. It requires a thorough knowledge of food microbiology (an important discipline in itself), and the training of all staff in aspects of hygiene. Consumers are demanding better products, yet numbers of recorded cases of foodborne disease and food poisoning continue to rise. We must diligently use all available information to ensure that consumers receive food that is of the standard of quality and safety that they have a right to expect.

Bibliography and references

General bibliography

1. Board, R.G. (1983) *A Modern Introduction to Food Microbiology*. Oxford: Blackwell. 0 632 00165 8
2. Cliver, D.O. (ed.) (1990) *Foodborne Diseases*. San Diego: Academic Press. 0 12 176558 X
3. Doyle, M.P. (ed.) (1989) *Foodborne Bacterial Pathogens*. New York: Marcel Dekker. 0 8247 778669
4. Felix, C.W. (ed.) (1987) *Food Protection Technology*. Michigan: Lewis. 0 87371 047 9
5. Harrigan, W.F. & McCance, M.E. (1976) *Laboratory Methods in Food and Dairy Microbiology*. London: Academic Press. 0 12 326040 X
6. Herschdoerfer, S.M. (ed.) (1984–1987) *Quality Control in the Food Industry*, 2nd edn. 4 vols. London: Academic Press. 0 12 343001 1, 0 12 343002 X, 0 12 343003 8, 0 12 343004 6.
7. Hobbs, B.C. & Roberts, D. (1987) *Food Poisoning and Food Hygiene*, 5th edn. London: Edward Arnold. 0 7131 4516 1
8. International Commission on Microbiological Specifications for Foods (ICMSF): *Microorganisms in Foods* (1978) *Vol. 1: Their Significance and Methods of Enumeration*, 2nd edn. Toronto: University of Toronto Press. 0 8020 2293 6
9. ICMSF: *Microorganisms in Foods* (1986) *Vol. 2: Sampling for Microbiological Analysis: Principles and Specific Applications*. Oxford: Blackwell. 0 632 01567 5
10. ICMSF: *Microorganisms in Foods* (1980) *Microbial Ecology of Foods*, 2 vols. New York: Academic Press. 0 12 363501 2, 0 12 363502 0
11. ICMSF: *Microorganisms in Foods* (1988) *Vol. 4: Application of the Hazard Analysis Critical Control Point (HACCP) System to Ensure Microbiological Safety and Quality*. Oxford: Blackwell. 0 632 02181 0

12. Jay, J.M. (1986) *Modern Food Microbiology*, 3rd edn. New York: Van Nostrand Reinhold. 0 442 24445 2
13. Mossel, D.A.A. (1982) *Microbiology of Foods*, 3rd edn. Utrecht: University of Utrecht. 90 6159 007 8
14. National Research Council Subcommittee on Microbiological Criteria (1985) *An Evaluation of the Role of Microbiological Criteria for Foods and Food Ingredients*. Washington DC: National Academy Press. 0 309 03497 3
15. Pierson, M.D. & Stern, N.J. (1986) *Foodborne Microorganisms and Their Toxins: Developing Methodology*. New York: Marcel Dekker. 0 8247 7607 0
16. Society for Applied Bacteriology Symposium Series Number 11: Roberts, T.A. & Skinner, F.A. (eds) (1983) *Food Microbiology: Advances and Prospects*. London: Academic Press. 0 12 589670 0
17. Sutherland, J.P., Varnam, A.H. & Evans, M.G. (1986) *A Colour Atlas of Food Quality Control*. London: Wolfe. 0 723 408157

Chapter bibliography and references

Chapter 1

Refs 1, 12 and:

Brock, T.D. & Madigan, M.T. (1991) *Biology of Microorganisms*, 6th edn. Englewood Cliffs: Prentice Hall. 0 13 086604 0
Davis, B.D., Dulbecco, R., Eisen, H.N. & Ginsberg, H.S. (1990) *Microbiology*, 4th edn. Philadelphia: J.B. Lippincott. 0 397 50689 9
Stanier, R.Y., Ingraham, J.L., Wheelis, M.L. & Painter, P.R. (1987) *General Microbiology*, 5th edn. Basingstoke: Macmillan. 0 333 41768 2

Chapter 2

Refs 2, 3 and:

Christensen, M.L. (1989) Human viral gastroenteritis. *Clinical Microbiology Reviews* **2**: 51–89.
Davis, B.D., Dulbecco, R., Eisen, H.N. & Ginsberg, H.S. (1990) *Microbiology*, 4th edn. Philadelphia: J.B. Lippincott. 0 397 50689 9
Griffith, P.L. & Park, R.W.A. (1990) Campylobacters associated with human diarrhoeal disease. *Journal of Applied Bacteriology* **69**: 281–301.
House of Commons Agriculture Committee (1990) *Fifth Report: Bovine Spongiform Encephalopathy (BSE)*. London: HMSO. 0 10 244990 2

Chapter 3

Refs 2, 3, 5 and:

Hardt-English, P., York, G., Stier, R. & Cocotas, P. (1990) Staphylococcal food poisoning outbreaks caused by canned mushrooms from China. *Food Technology* **44**: 74–77.
Moreau, C. (1974) *Moulds, Toxins and Food*. (Translated and edited by M.O. Moss). Chichester: John Wiley. 0 471 99681 5
Wood, G.M. *et al.* (1990) Studies on a toxic metabolite from the mould *Wallemia*. *Food Additives and Contaminants* **7**: 69–77.

Chapter 4

Refs 2, 3, 5 and:

Janda, J.M., Powers, C., Bryant, R.G. & Abbott, S.L. (1988) Current perspectives on the epidemiology and pathogenesis of clinically significant *Vibrio* spp. *Clinical Microbiology Reviews* **1**: 245–267.
Karmali, M.A. (1989) Infection by verocytotoxin-producing *Escherichia coli*. *Clinical Microbiology Reviews* **2**: 15–38.
PHLS (1990a) Laboratory diagnosis of infection caused by Vero cytotoxin-producing *Escherichia coli* of serogroup O157. *Public Health Laboratory Digest* **7** (4): 94–95.
PHLS (1990b) Vero cytotoxin-producing *Escherichia coli* O157. Proceedings of a Seminar, London, 1 June 1990. *Public Health Laboratory Digest* **7** (4, Supplement): 116–170.

Chapter 5

Refs 1, 12, 16, 17 and:

Dainty, R.H. (1985) Bacterial growth in food, a nutrient-rich environment. *Special Publications of the Society for General Microbiology*, **16**: *Bacteria in their Natural Environments* (eds M. Fletcher & G.D. Floodgate) pp. 171–188. London: Academic Press. 0 12 260561 6
Mossel, D.A.A. & Ingram, M. (1955) The physiology of the microbial spoilage of foods. *Journal of Applied Bacteriology* **18**: 232–268.

Chapter 6

Refs 10, 12 and:

Gould, G.W. (ed.) (1989) *Mechanisms of Action of Food Preservation Procedures*. London: Elsevier Applied Science. 1 85166 293 6
Roberts, T.A. *et al.* (eds) (1981) *Psychrotrophic Microorganisms in Spoilage and Pathogenicity*. London: Academic Press. 0 12 589720 0
Rockland, L.B. & Beuchat, L.R. (1987) *Water Activity: Theory & Applications to Food*. New York: Marcel Dekker. 0 8247 7759 X
Society for Applied Bacteriology Technical Series. No. 13: Russell, A.D. & Fuller, R. (eds) (1979) *Cold Tolerant Microbes in Spoilage and the Environment*. London: Academic Press. 0 12 603750 7
Society for Applied Bacteriology Technical Series, No. 15: Gould, G.W. & Corry, J.E.L. (1980) *Microbial Growth in Extremes of Environment*. London: Academic Press. 0 12 293680 9
Troller, J.A. & Christian, J.H.B. (1978) *Water Activity and Food*. New York: Academic Press. 0 12 700650 8

Chapter 7

Refs 10, 12 and:

Branen, A.L. & Davidson, P.M. (eds) (1983) *Antimicrobials in Foods*. New York: Marcel Dekker. 0 8247 7026 9
Cerf, O. (1977) Tailing of survival curves of bacterial spores. *Journal of Applied Bacteriology* **42**: 1–19.
Gould, G.W. (ed.) (1989) *Mechanisms of Action of Food Preservation Procedures*. London: Elsevier Applied Science. 1 85166 293 6
Moats, W.A. (1971a) Kinetics of thermal death of bacteria. *Journal of Bacteriology* **105**: 165–171.
Moats, W.A. (1971b) Interpretation of nonlogarithmic survivor curves of heated bacteria. *Journal of Food Science* **36**: 523–526.
Pethybridge, A.D., Ison, R.W. & Harrigan, W.F. (1983) Dissociation constant of sorbic acid in water and water–glycerol mixtures at 25°C from conductance measurements. *Journal of Food Technology* **18**: 789–796.
Stumbo, C.R. (1973) *Thermobacteriology in Food Processing*, 2nd edn. New York: Academic Press. 0 12 7200769 2
Urbain, W.M. (1986) *Food Irradiation*. Orlando: Academic Press. 0 12 709370 2

Chapter 8

Refs 4, 14, laws and statutes as listed in the text, and:

Brown, S.A. (1989) General principles of regulation: foods and beverages. In *International Food Regulation Handbook* (ed. R.D. Middlekauff & P. Shubik). New York: Marcel Dekker. 0 8247 7909 6
Carpenter, J. & Whitington, R. (1419) *Liber Albus: The White Book of the City of London*. (Translated by H.T. Riley, 1861.) London: R. Griffin.

Chapter 9

Various ISO and BS standards as listed in the text and:

HMSO (1989) *Chilled and Frozen: Guidelines in Cook–Chill and Cook–Freeze Catering Systems*. London: HMSO. 0 11 321161 9
IFST (1987) *Food and Drink Manufacture: Good Manufacturing Practice – A Guide to its Responsible Management*. London: The Institute of Food Science & Technology (UK). 0 905367 02 2
IFST (1990) *Guidelines for the Handling of Chilled Foods*, 2nd edn. London: The Institute of Food Science & Technology (UK). 0 905367 07 3
Oakland, J.S. (1989) *Total Quality Management*. Oxford: Heinemann. 0 89397 348 3

Chapter 10

Various ISO, BSI and EC standards as indicated in the text and:

Park, R.W.A. (1990) Joint IUMS/ICFMH and UNESCO consultation on postgraduate teaching in advanced food microbiology with recommendation of a core curriculum. *International Journal of Food Microbiology* **11**: 107–118.
Skovsgaard, N. (1990) The need for continuous training in food factories. *International Journal of Food Microbiology* **11**: 119–126.

Chapter 11

Advisory Committee on Dangerous Pathogens (1990) *Categorization of Pathogens According to Hazard and Categories of Containment*, 2nd edn. London: HMSO. 0 11 885564 6
Clark, R.P. *et al.* (1990) Open fronted safety cabinets in ventilated laboratories. *Journal of Applied Bacteriology* **69**: 338–358.
Collins, C.H. (1988) *Laboratory-acquired Infections: History, Incidence, Causes and Prevention*, 2nd edn. London: Butterworths. 0 40 700218 9

Miller, B.M. (ed.) (1986) *Laboratory Safety: Principles and Practices*. Washington, DC: American Society for Microbiology. 0 914826 77 8

Chapter 12

Refs 5, 8, 13, 15, various ISO and BSI standards as indicated in the text and:

Futter, B.V. & Richardson, G. (1971) Anaerobic jars in the quantitative recovery of clostridia. In *Isolation of Anaerobes* (eds D.A. Shapton & R.G. Board) *Society for Applied Bacteriology Technical Series* **5**. London: Academic Press.

Karmali, M.A. (1989) Infection by verocytotoxin-producing *Escherichia coli*. *Clinical Microbiology Reviews* **2**: 15–38.

PHLS (1990a) Laboratory diagnosis of infection caused by Vero cytotoxin-producing *Escherichia coli* of serogroup O157. *Public Health Laboratory Digest* **7** (4): 94–95.

PHLS (1990b) Vero cytotoxin-producing *Escherichia coli* O157. Proceedings of a Seminar, London, 1 June 1990. *Public Health Laboratory Digest* **7** (4, Supplement): 116–170.

Silverstolpe, L. *et al.* (1961) An epidemic among infants caused by *Salmonella muenchen*. *Journal of Applied Bacteriology* **24**: 134–142.

Society for Applied Bacteriology Symposium Series, No. 12: Andrew, M.H.E. & Russell, A.D. (eds) (1984) *The Revival of Injured Microbes*. London: Academic Press. 0 12 058520 0

Society for Applied Bacteriology Technical Series, No. 17: Corry, J.E.L., Roberts, D. & Skinner, F.A. (eds) (1982) *Isolation and Identification Methods for Food Poisoning Organisms*. London: Academic Press. 0 12 189950 0

Chapter 13

Ref. 15 and:

Firstenberg-Eden, R. & Eden, G. (1984) *Impedance Microbiology*. New York: Wiley. 0 471 90623 9

Pettipher, G.L. (1983) *The Direct Epifluorescent Filter Technique for the Rapid Enumeration of Micro-organisms*. Letchworth: Research Studies Press. 0 86380 607 6

Sharpe, A.N. & Peterkin, P.I. (1988) *Membrane Filter Food Microbiology*. New York: Wiley. 0 471 91790 7

Society for Applied Bacteriology Technical Series, No. 24: Grange, J.M., Fox, A. & Morgan, N.L. (eds) *Immunological Techniques in Microbiology*. Oxford: Blackwell. 0 632 01908 5

Society for Applied Bacteriology Technical Series, No. 25: Stannard, C.J., Petitt, S.B. & Skinner, F.A. (eds) *Rapid Microbiological Methods for Foods, Beverages and Pharmaceuticals*. Oxford: Blackwell. 0 632 02629 4

Society for Applied Bacteriology Technical Series, No. 26: Stanley, P.E., McCarthy, B.J. & Smither, R. (eds) *ATP Luminescence*. Oxford: Blackwell. 0 632 02716 9

Chapter 14

Refs 4, 5, 9, 14 and:

Duncan, A.J. (1965) *Quality Control and Industrial Statistics*, 3rd edn. Homewood, Ill: Irwin. 65012414

Smelt, J.P.P.M. & Quadt, J.F.A. (1990) A proposal for using previous experience in designing microbiological sampling plans based on variables. *Journal of Applied Bacteriology* **69**: 504–511.

Wetherill, G.B. (1977) *Sampling Inspection and Quality Control*, 2nd edn. London: Chapman & Hall. 0 412 14960 5

Chapter 15

Ref. 5 and:

Best, D.J. (1990) Optimal determination of most probable numbers. *International Journal of Food Microbiology* **11**: 159–166.

Cochran, W.G. (1950) Estimation of bacterial densities by means of the 'most probable number'. *Biometrics* **6**: 105–116.

de Man, J.C. (1975) The probability of most probable numbers. *European Journal of Applied Microbiology* **1**: 67–78.

de Man, J.C. (1977) MPN tables for more than one test. *European Journal of Applied Microbiology* **4**: 307–316.

Duncan, A.J. (1965) *Quality Control and Industrial Statistics*, 3rd edn. Homewood, Ill: Irwin. 65012414

Lucas, J.M. (1973) A modified 'V' mask control scheme. *Technometrics* **15**: 833–847.

Lucas, J.M. (1976) The design and use of V-mask control schemes. *Journal of Quality Technology* **8**: 1–12.

Lucas, J.M. (1982) Combined Shewhart–CUSUM quality control schemes. *Journal of Quality Technology* **14**: 51–59.

Oakland, J.S. & Followell, R.F. (1990) *Statistical Process Control*, 2nd edn. Oxford: Heinemann. 0 434 91484 3

Ryan, T.P. (1989) *Statistical Methods for Quality Improvement*. London: John Wiley. 0 471 84337 7

Tillett, H.E. (1987) Most probable numbers of organisms: revised tables for the multiple tube method. *Epidemiology and Infection* **99**: 471–476.

Wetherill, G.B. (1977) *Sampling Inspection and Quality Control*, 2nd edn. London: Chapman & Hall. 0 412 14960 5

Woodward, R.L. (1957) How probable is the most probable number? *Journal of the American Water Works Association* **49**: 1060ff.

Chapter 16

Refs 4, 10, 11, 14 and:

Committee on the Microbiological Safety of Food (1990) *The Microbiological Safety of Food* ('The Richmond Report') Parts 1 and 2. London: HMSO. Part 1, 0 11 321273 9, Part 2, 0 11 321347 6

Mayes, T. & Kilsby, D.C. (1989) The use of HAZOP hazard analysis to identify critical control points for the microbiological safety of food. *Food Quality and Preference* **1**: 53–57.

Mossel, D.A.A. & Ingram, M. (1955) The physiology of the microbial spoilage of foods. *Journal of Applied Bacteriology* **18**: 232–268.

Mossel, D.A.A. & van Netten, P. (1990) *Staphylococcus aureus* and related staphylococci in foods: ecology, proliferation, toxigenesis, control and monitoring. *Journal of Applied Bacteriology* **69** (**Symposium Supplement**), 123S–145S.

Index